The Gift Of An Open Heart

The Gift Of An Open Heart

the struggle from birth to graduation
for a young heart patient

by Nicholas Zerwas

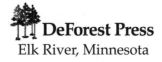

DeForest Press
Elk River, Minnesota

Permission gratefully acknowledged for photos and articles from Star News, ECM
Publishers, Inc.

Published by:
DeForest Press
P.O. Box 154
Elk River, MN 55330 USA
www.DeForestPress.com
Phone: 763-428-2997
Toll-free: 877-441-9733
Richard DeForest Erickson, Publisher
Shane Groth, President

Cover design by Linda Walters, Optima Graphics, Appleton, WI

ISBN 1-930374-17-8

Library of Congress Cataloging-in-Publication Data

Zerwas, Nick, 1980-
  The gift of an open heart : the struggle from birth to graduation for a young heart
patient / by Nick Zerwas.
     p. cm.
  ISBN 1-930374-17-8
1. Zerwas, Nick, 1980---Health. 2. Heart--Surgery--Patients--Minnesota--Biography.
3. Congenital heart disease in children--Surgery. I. Title.
  RJ426.C64Z47 2005
  362.197'412'0092--dc22

                            2005019643

I would like to dedicate this book and my story to the children and families my parents and I were blessed enough to meet during our stays at Minneapolis Children's Hospital. Many of these children were much sicker than I was and lived very intense, but sadly short lives. Their strength through their sickness and their determination to live life fully while at death's doorstep continue to drive me to never waste a day of my gift of life. While there are too many children to possibly name all of them, my little buddy Blake certainly stands out.

Blake was born while I was waiting for a heart transplant. His heart defect was very serious, but he was a strong and brave little boy. It was hard not to look at him with his blonde hair and smile, and not picture myself at his age going through the same challenges. Maybe that's why news of his passing hurt so deep, but whatever the reason, when he was gone my heart was broken.

Like many chronically ill children with a zest for life and a spirit that can't be dampened, just a few years of life was all he needed to change everyone he came into contact with. Blake, along with the other children and families I met at Minneapolis Children's Hospital, have influenced me beyond imagination, and for that I will be forever grateful.

Nick Zerwas was the most memorable student that I worked with in my school career of almost 40 years. Nick was a student that was always on the verge of a medical crisis, yet he performed as well as any student in school. Nick could of felt sorry for himself and let others wait on him hand and foot. His attitude was to do as much for himself as possible without whining or complaining.

I probably knew Nick as well as I knew any student. Nick, Chuck Schuldt, Ryan Ebert and I had lunch together every Friday.

Nick was a member of the National Honor Society, Student Council and was the student representative to the VandenBerge Site Council. Nick's enthusiasm and positive attitude were contagious. Nick used a wheel chair to get around only to get more done in a shorter time.

I remember his insight and sense of humor. On one occasion he was sitting in the office with his feet on the desk and I was complaining about the work that was piling up. Nick looked over at me and said, "Gaarder, instead of complaining, why don't you take one item from the pile, finish it, and then you will have one less thing to do."

Nick was interested in politics even as a junior high student. Our Friday lunches were called meetings of the Sherburne County Republican Party and the office was designated as the Republican Party Headquarters. In the last Minnesota election Nick was close to being selected as the Republican Candidate for State Senate, the seat held by Mike Jungbauer.

Nick has accomplished more by the age of 24 than most people do in a life span of 60 years. One can only speculate on his achievements if he had been given normal health.

Ronald E. Gaarder
Principal, VandenBerg Jr. High School, retired

Contents

Foreword

It is said that as parents we learn from our children and as teachers we learn from our students. Certainly it follows that the physician-patient relationship facilitates learning as well. In my almost twenty-five year relationship with Nicholas Zerwas, it has been my privilege to have learned a great deal from this remarkable young man.

Nick's story is not in and of itself unique, for indeed almost every individual with a chronic medical condition has a potentially compelling story to tell. However, I think that the reader will quickly recognize that Nick's story is indeed special. By virtue of tremendous strength of character, wit, wisdom, and a maturity that always far exceeded his chronologic age, Nick invariably met the numerous challenges of his medical condition with grace and dignity. He was always positive and upbeat even in the face of formidable obstacles. What I believe is special about his story is how Nick genuinely enriched the life of all those with whom he came to know during his remarkable journey.

Undoubtedly Nick, like others of his generation, has benefited immeasurably from the advances in the treatment of congenital heart defects that have occurred over the last quarter century. Numerous health care providers have been participants in Nick's care, but I would be remiss if I did not mention one in particular—the late Dr. Demetre M. Nicoloff. Dr. Nicoloff was a friend, mentor, and colleague. He was a gifted and compassionate cardiac surgeon, and over the years, the "two Nicks," patient and surgeon, developed a special relationship as well.

As students of medicine, one can be taught the scientific aspect of patient care in the classroom and laboratory, but the art of medicine is learned from our patients, and I am forever grateful for Nick as a teacher.

I trust that the reader will be enriched by sharing in Nick Zerwas's story, and I sense that we likely will hear more of his story in the future as Nick's journey continues.

FREDERIC M. STONE, MD

Acknowledgments

This book would not be possible without the help, support and encouragement of many people. Richard Erickson and Shane Groth of DeForest Press provided the experience and guidance I needed to launch such an endeavor. Without their help this certainly would not have been possible.

Throughout my life my family and I have been blessed with angels in our lives. The constant support provided to us by friends, extended family, and oftentimes complete strangers made it possible for us to make it through the challenges we faced as a family.

The unbounded enthusiasm of my teachers to keep me involved in school and caught up in my classes is what made it possible for me to graduate with my class. Their support and encouragement kept me motivated even when things looked bleak. I truly appreciated the extra effort from all of the teachers willing to go the extra mile to help me succeed. These teachers and administrators include, but are not limited to: Wayne Stensgard, my sixth grade teacher; Doug Bloom, my ninth grade geometry teacher; Carol Erickson, my ninth grade English teacher; Dave Conley, my ninth grade health teacher; Ron Gaarder and Jim Weinman, my junior high school principals; Ken Jordan and James Voight, my senior high administrators.

There are few people who can say that their best friend on graduation day, is the same person they were best friends with as a toddler. Ryan Ebert has been in my life through nearly as many surgeries as have my own parents. He and his family supported my family through all of the uncertain times and were there to celebrate with us after each success. It takes a special person to be willing to put the needs of their friend ahead of themselves throughout all of elementary, junior high, and high school. Every day in junior high and high school, Ryan gave up the usual social time between classes to pick me up from my class, push me across the school to my next class, and then hustle to his own. Ryan's love and friendship is something that I continue to cherish and appreciate to this day.

Countless doctors and nurses have dedicated their careers to insure that myself and other sick children like me always received the best possible medical care. Of course I would like to specifically recognize my cardiologist, Dr. Frederic Stone, and my heart surgeon, the late Dr. Demetre Nicoloff. Along with being an amazing cardiologist, Dr. Stone is an amazing and kind person. He is the exact kind of man every patient would want at their side. Dr. Nicoloff was an unbelievably gifted doctor, but he was probably the most humble human being I have ever met in my life.

My grandparents, my parents, and my two brothers, David, Tommy, and his wife Karla, were always at my side offering their unwavering love and support. They put their lives on hold and oftentimes focused their time and energy on making sure I was well. There should be no doubt that without them I would not have had the strength to keep fighting.

My high school sweetheart, and now my wife, Julie, provides me with the strength and confidence I use to carry myself through everyday. She pushes me to be the best, almost as much as I push myself, and for that I am very grateful. Her intense love and devotion inspires me everyday to make the most of our new life together.

It All Begins With The Heart

"Mom, I have been working on this speech for a week," I half-heartedly complained. "Can you help me out a little bit?"

My mom walked from the kitchen into the dining room and stood over me as I sat at the dining room table. "Nick, you wanted to be senior class president, and now you have to write a speech for graduation. I didn't run for senior class president," she teased.

"I know, I know...can you just help me with the wording of a few things?" I asked in my most desperate voice.

She sat down next to me and began reading what I had written down. I watched her lips move as she read the words, and I beamed as she read over some of the lines I was particularly proud of.

"You know, I just can't believe we're finally here," she said with an emotional pause. "You're graduating! I just can't believe we made it...eighteen years ago I would have never thought either of us would make it." Her voice trailed off as she went back to reading.

"It's a boy!" the doctor announced. He wrapped the bundled baby up in several blankets and presented him to his proud parents.

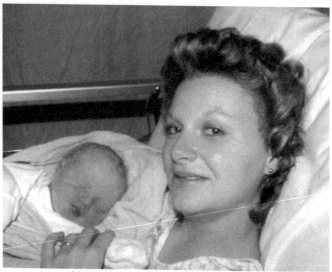

Mom with Nick, born December 15, 1980

"Ten fingers and ten toes!" Tom announced, assuring his wife that their baby was healthy and normal.

Tom and Chris were excited with the thought of having a baby around the house again. When Nick was three days old Chris began getting things in order to pack up and prepare for the trip home. Before her baby was ready to be discharged from Mercy Hospital he underwent a circumcision.

As the doctor completed the circumcision Chris was surprised when she heard the doctors raising their voices.

"Oxygen, I need an O2 mask over here!" one doctor barked.

There was confusion and panic throughout the room as doctors and nurses began rushing in every direction. Chris yelled for her husband, "Tom! Tom! What's going on? What's happening?"

Tom went to his wife's side and attempted to comfort her. The head doctor quickly regained control of the situation and continued to deliver orders to a waiting army of doctors and nurses. "Get him on oxygen and call Children's and tell them

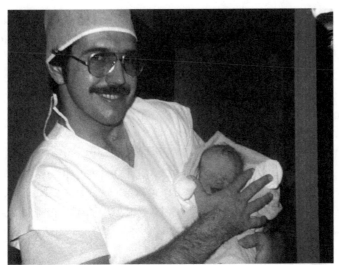

Dad and newborn Nick

we will have one enroute," he ordered. "Call downstairs and ready an ambulance. Lets go! We need to do this quickly!"

Tom looked in between two doctors frantically working on his son, Nick. He was horrified when he saw that his son had turned a dark, bluish-purple in color. Tom hugged his wife and prayed for everything to be okay.

Chris was nearing a level of hysteria as she saw the nurses begin to wheel her son out of her hospital room. "Where are you taking him? Where is he going? Please, someone tell me what's happening!" she pleaded with the nurses.

Finally, a nurse grabbed both Tom and Chris and pulled them into a corner of the hospital room. As Nick was wheeled out of the room, the doctor who had been working on him the most walked across the room towards Tom and Chris. He began speaking, "Mr. and Mrs. Zerwas, my name is Dr. ..."

"Where are they taking my son?" Chris demanded as she cut the doctor off in mid sentence. "What is going on? What happened? Where is my baby going?"

"Okay, Nick is being transferred to Minneapolis Children's Hospital. Once he arrives he will be evaluated by several specialists to determine what the problem is."

"What happened? Why did my son turn blue? Is he alive? Is he breathing?" Tom asked rapidly. "And where is he now? Should one of us be with him? Can we ride with him to the other hospital?"

"Your son is alive. He is still breathing, but I don't know what's wrong with him. Once he arrives at Minneapolis Children's Hospital they will began some tests to determine what the problem is. As far as the ambulance goes, you two will have to follow it to Minneapolis. There will be too many people inside working on the baby."

As the ambulance quickly left with sirens screaming, Tom and Chris shuddered and attempted to regain their bearings.

Tom followed the ambulance as best he could. As they reached traffic the ambulance weaved through the cars ahead flawlessly, while Tom did his best to stay on the road. Chris sat in the passenger seat of the station wagon, her mind racing. She didn't really understand what had happened, and how her family was going to make it through this. As the ambulance carrying Nick pulled out of sight ahead of them, Chris wondered if she would ever see her baby alive again. Tom and Chris didn't quite know what to say during the ride to the hospital, so neither of them said hardly anything. Tom wiped tears from his cheeks and cleared his throat loudly. Chris slumped over and softly cried to herself.

By the time they arrived to the hospital, Nick had already been admitted through the emergency room and transferred into the pediatric intensive care unit. As they walked through the door into the emergency room they both supported each other. They leaned in, each using the other one to stay upright. A tall, thin man with thick, curly hair was standing in the doorway. Tom and Chris stopped and looked around trying to determine where to go to find their son.

The thin man approached Tom and Chris and introduced himself. "Hello, I am Dr. Frederic Stone. I am a pediatric cardiologist. I am taking care of Nicholas," he told them with an intense look on his face. Dr. Stone escorted Tom and Chris to a private room and began explaining what he knew about Nick.

"Mr. and Mrs. Zerwas...I have some news that will be difficult for you to hear."

With that Chris began crying again, and Tom held her closely. Dr. Stone continued, "Your son Nicholas is not the healthy baby you thought he was. Nick was actually born with a very rare and serious heart defect."

"Oh my God," Chris gasped, as Tom put his head into his hands and began crying.

Dr. Stone pressed on, "Nick was born with a heart defect called Tricuspid Atresia, and it is gravely serious. We will need to do two open-heart surgeries fairly early on, and hopefully those surgeries will allow his heart to pump enough oxygen for his body to sustain itself."

"What happens after that?" Chris blurted out. "After those surgeries will everything be okay?"

"Well, those surgeries will allow Nick to live several years; however, even with all the advancements of medical science your son will not live past seven years of age," Dr. Stone said as he leaned forward and looked into his hands resting on his lap.

"Oh, NO, NO, NO" Chris cried. "No, please, please don't say that!" Tom looked up with tears blurring his vision, and reached out to hug his wife. They sat holding each other, and as they both calmed down, Tom asked, "What are we going to do? How do we get through this?"

Dr. Stone looked at them and said, "By relying on each other and doing the best you can. There are two ways this can go. Either this will strengthen your marriage and make your family closer than you ever thought possible, or this will destroy your marriage, your family, and your lives. You need to work together to survive this."

Tom and Chris looked at Dr. Stone and listened to him intently. They held each other's hands tightly, and promised to make it through this together. Chris thanked Dr. Stone for his help and support. "Could you explain our son's heart defect again," asked Tom, "and how it is different from a regular heart."

"Nick was born with effectively a three-chambered heart, instead of a regular four-chambered heart. Nick's heart is missing the right ventricle, which normally pumps the blood to the lungs. So, Nick's heart has a unique blood flow with the absence of the right atrium. Blood is mixing in the left side of Nick's heart and being pumped to the lungs and the body both by the left ventricle. This mixing of blood is causing a lack of oxygen and is the source of Nick's bluish color and cardiac symptoms."

Dr. Stone left Tom and Chris in that small conference room, and as they gathered themselves they promised each other to listen to Dr. Stone's advice and work on making it through this together. Chris and Tom took up vigil along their baby's bedside in the intensive care unit at Minneapolis Children's Hospital. Chris stayed with her son in the hospital the entire time. She only left his side a few times each day to go into the basement of the hospital to the room designated for smokers. Tom traveled to the hospital each afternoon after work and stayed late into the night.

On the afternoon of December 24, Tom and Chris were finally able to bring their son, Nicholas, named after the patron saint of children, home from the hospital. When they finally had him home, however, they immediately thought of bringing him back to the hospital, where they knew he would be safe. The first nights were restless as their colicky baby with blue lips and ash-gray complexion cried until he lost consciousness.

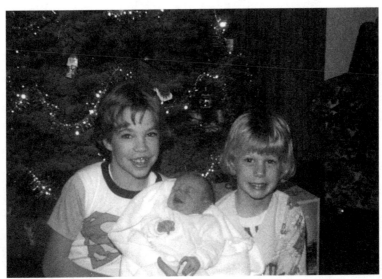

Nick with brothers Tommy (left) and David (right), Christmas 1980

Chris sobbed as she held what she thought was her dead baby in her arms.

Middle of the night trips down to Children's Hospital was the rule rather then the exception. The doctors struggled to understand how or why the baby would not stop crying before he passed out. Whatever the problem was, the doctors decided the first surgery had to be done earlier then anticipated. With their baby just two months old, Tom and Chris drove to the hospital to bring Nick in for his first open heart surgery.

The First
Open Heart Surgery

Chris rocked back and forth, clutching her baby in her arms. She softly sobbed as Tom gently rubbed her back, trying in vain to provide some comfort. As they huddled together they took turns kissing their child. Suddenly the door to the private waiting area opened, and the doctor who introduced himself earlier as the person who would be putting their child to sleep entered the room.

The doctor drew in a long deep breath and said, "Okay, Tom and Chris, I am here for Nick." Still crying, Tom carried his already sleeping child over to the doctor and placed his son into the doctor's arms.

Chris wept, "Please, please don't let anything happen to my baby."

Time seemed to stand still for Tom and Chris. The waiting was more difficult than they could have imagined. They sat together and waited, along with other family members. Their brothers and sisters and friends waited with them holding constant vigil in the hospital waiting room. Nurses commented they had never seen so much family for a single patient.

Dr. Stone appeared in the doorway to the waiting room and confidently walked across the room. He sat down next to Chris and Tom and began discussing the surgery. "The operation appears to have been successful," he said. "Your child is alive." Tom and Chris hugged Dr. Stone and continued to weep, thanking him for saving their child. They then announced the good news to the family and friends in the waiting room.

Tom and Chris looked around the intensive care unit; the hum of ventilators and the beeping of heart monitors filled the unit. After spending nearly a week in the ICU with Nick shortly after he was born, they had become accustomed to the constant sounds of the hospital. Looking at their child laying motionless in the hospital bed, they both knew this hospital stay was going to be very different than the others. Nick was unconscious and not yet breathing on his own. A ventilator was connected to a breathing tube inserted in Nick's trachea. The ventilator whooshed loudly as the machine breathed for the two-month-old. Chest tubes draining fluid were protruding from their baby's heavily bandaged chest. Their son didn't appear to have any life of his own left in him. Chris sat in the chair next to her baby's bed, yearning to hold him. She rubbed his tiny foot, one of the only parts of her child that wasn't occupied by a wire, tube, or bandage.

The days in the hospital grew long and tiresome. Chris slept in a closet-like room adjacent to the ICU, on a chair that folded semi-flat. She would wake early to clean up in the restroom, and then walk to her son's bedside to sit with him for the day. A constant stream of doctors, nurses, and surgeons would file in throughout the day to check on Nick's condition. Chris was always at her son's side listening to those who were treating Nick. When doctors visited, Chris insisted on being updated on Nick's condition. She soon became a quasi-expert on cardiac function, and the treatments for lowering fluid retention and increasing cardiac output.

By late afternoon as the flow of doctors through the room slowed, Tom arrived at the hospital, coming directly from work. Chris immediately updated Tom on all of the progress made in the day, along with the encouraging words of the doctors and nurses. Tom used this time at the hospital to be with Nick and to support his wife. He often brought their other two children to the hospital.

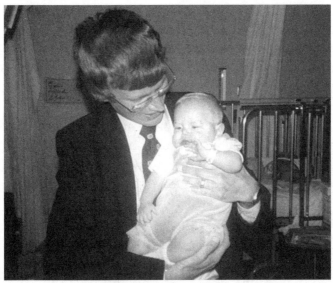
Nick and Dr. Stone, 1981

Tommy and David loved going to the hospital with their dad and seeing their little brother and their mom. The boys stayed with neighbors and relatives often and loved any chance they got to be with both of their parents. When they were staying away from their parents they told anyone who would listen about their brave brother. They constantly talked about how strong their brother was, and how he had his heart operated on. At the hospital, Tommy and David loved reading stories out loud to Nick. When they weren't reading to him they would talk to him, telling him absolutely everything that happened to them since the last time they were able to visit.

As the weeks passed, Nick's recovery began to steadily progress. Nick fought off and overcame battles with pneumonia and other all too common infections patients tend to come in contact with in the hospital. Soon the ventilator was removed and Nick was breathing on his own. Chris was able to hear her baby crying from the bank of parent sleeping rooms, which was strangely comforting to her. As Nick's hospital stay began to wind down, Chris was looking forward to bringing her son home. She was also a bit nervous about Nick being home, however, where his blood pressure and oxygen levels wouldn't be constantly monitored. The nurses reassured her, as always, and gave her the confidence she needed to feel like she could handle Nick at home.

Nearly six weeks after Tom and Chris brought Nick in for heart surgery, they were finally bringing their son home. It would also be Chris's first trip home since Nick was admitted for the operation. As they pulled in the driveway to their home, with Nick strapped into his car seat in the back of the station wagon, Tom and Chris noticed a large banner draped across the front of their home. A giant placard reading, WELCOME HOME! spanned nearly the entire width of the garage. Their families, friends and neighbors soon poured out of their home to welcome them and to celebrate the successful surgery.

Nick was still extremely sick, even after the successful surgery. He was small, even for a five-month-old, and was not very active. His color was still very poor. Nick's complexion was very ash colored, his lips were a dark purple color, and his finger and toenails had a deep blue coloring. Nick's heart was still not pumping the oxygen his little body demanded. The nearly constant lack of oxygen severely hampered Nick's growth and stunted his cognitive developments. As the months passed Nick's health continued to neither thrive nor fail, he simply maintained.

Chris and Tom took Nick for his eighteen-month-old appointment with a new pediatrician at a clinic in town. The doctor visited with them and was very interested in Nick's heart condition and the surgery done at Children's Hospital. She asked Chris about Nick's eating and sleeping habits. She inquired about the level of physical activity Nick engaged in regularly. Chris informed the doctor that as of yet Nick was not walking; he was not even crawling. At eighteen months old, Nick was not even rolling over in his crib.

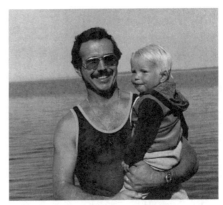

Nick and Dad at beach, 1982

The pediatrician was very discouraged by this revelation, and suggested that maybe it was time to discuss what these signs were indicating. She told Tom and Chris that this physical and cognitive delay in Nick's development indicated that something besides his heart condition was occurring. She then looked at both of them and mater of factly said, "Well, Chris, Tom, it looks like you need to start preparing yourself for mental retardation."

Chris screamed and shook, and she abruptly stood and picked up Nick, who was still strapped into his car seat. Tom sat in his chair not saying a word, his face becoming hot and flushed. When he gathered himself he stood, opened the door to the hallway, and abruptly left. Chris followed Tom out of the office carrying Nick in his carrier, and they drove directly to Dr. Stone's office in Children's Hospital. As they sat in the waiting room Chris wiped at a constant stream of tears falling from her cheeks. Tom sat in the waiting room wanting to vomit, scream and cry all at the same time; instead, he sat there, hugged his wife, and told her everything was going to be okay.

Dr. Stone finished his previous appointment with another patient, and then asked his nurse to clear his afternoon schedule. Dr. Stone walked into the waiting room and greeted Tom and Chris with a long and comforting hug. He asked them to come into his office, where he immediately apologized for the comments made by the pediatrician. He explained that what she had said and done was not appropriate. Dr. Stone assured them that while Nick was certainly behind children his age, he was actually making remarkable progress. Chris somehow found the courage to ask, "Is Nick going to be mentally retarded?" Dr. Stone said, "Nick is behind. Will he always be behind? I don't know."

Chris held her son and softly cried. Dr. Stone reassured her that as Nick continued to make progress and as his health improved, he would begin to catch up developmentally with where he should be. Dr. Stone also told Tom and Chris that planning for Nick's second open heart surgery had already begun. The second surgery would be a shunt to direct more blood from the heart to the lungs. Dr. Stone explained that this surgery would be very similar to the other operation Nick had a little over a year earlier. Dr. Stone hoped this surgery would allow enough oxygen to be delivered to the body to fully meet the needs of Nick's body.

3
Year Two
Surgery Two

A few months later, for the second time in as many years, Tom and Chris carried their child into Minneapolis Children's hospital for open heart surgery. The waiting room again swelled with family and friends, all praying and hoping for good news. Tom and Chris waited in a private room for the anesthesiologist to again enter the room and take their child. Chris held Nick tightly in her arms, praying this wouldn't be the last time she held her child. Tom comforted his wife, even though he, too, was distraught at the idea of losing Nick.

Tommy sat on the far side of Chris and cried loudly into his mother's side, begging her not to let the doctors take Nick into surgery. David flanked the opposite side of his father and pleaded with him to keep Nick out of the hospital. Tommy and David were not old enough to really understand the necessity of the surgery. They only knew that the doctors were going to be doing a very risky surgery on their brother's heart.

As the family was locked in this bear hug-like huddle they all cried and hoped for the best. The huddle broke as the door to the private room opened and the doctor walked in. Knowing it was time, Tommy and David sobbed loudly and grabbed their

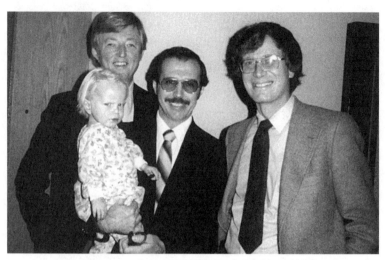

Dr. Bessenger (left), Nick, Tom (Dad), Dr. Stone (right)

parents tightly. Tom and Chris quietly stood and approached the anesthesiologist with their already sleeping child in their arms. They handed Nick to the doctor, and pleaded with him to watch over their son. Tom and Chris gathered their other two children and prepared for the long wait ahead of them.

As Nick's hospital bed was wheeled down the long hallway into surgery, Tom, Chris, and their two oldest boys walked into the main waiting area. The crowd of people who filled the room shocked Tom and Chris. Close family members were sitting next to distant cousins who were sitting next to friends and neighbors.

The number of people in the waiting area alarmed the nurses who walked by on their way to work. They were convinced a large-scale accident had occurred over night and that multiple patients were already in surgery. Nurses stared in disbelief as word passed that the crowd was for a single patient.

Tom and Chris appreciated the support of those who were waiting with them, but mainly kept to themselves. They split their time between the waiting room, the smoking area in the basement, and the hospital chapel. One of them always remained in the waiting room in case the doctor came out of surgery to give an update. Tommy and David passed the time by writing stories and coloring pictures for their little brother. They bragged to their aunts and uncles about their brother and how strong he was. They also showed off the pictures and stories they planned on decorating Nick's hospital room with.

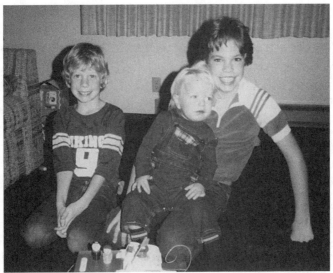

Nick with brothers David (left) and Tommy (right), Christmas 1982

When Dr. Stone finally entered the waiting room there was an unmistakable sense of confidence in his stride. He seemed to bound across the room as he approached Tom and Chris. Dr. Stone walked Tom and Chris into a private conference room and asked them to sit down. He explained the surgery was difficult, and the process of rerouting the blood through Nick's heart was very time consuming. However, he assured Tom and Chris that the surgery went well and it appeared to be successful. Dr. Stone cautioned Tom and Chris that Nick still wasn't breathing on his own, and that he was far from being out of the woods. Chris and Tom smiled as tears rolled down their cheeks. They hugged Dr. Stone and thanked him again for all that he had done for them.

Tom and Chris walked into the waiting room, gave their oldest children a hug, and told the crowd that Nick was out of surgery. They told everyone the doctors were optimistic about the surgery; however, Nick had a long road ahead of him. The crowd in the waiting room erupted in a cheer, and began hugging one another. Some of the people cried and others prayed. All of them were grateful. Tom and Chris thanked them for their continuing support and said they could not have survived this without them.

The all too familiar sounds of IV pumps and ventilator machines filled the intensive care unit as Tom and Chris walked through the doors of the unit. They followed Nick's nurse to a corner bed in the ICU separated from the neighboring bed by a thin curtain. The nurse explained that this open bay of beds was for the most critical patients. The patients were here in front of the nurses' station so they could be monitored by several nurses and doctors at all times.

Chris and Tom saw the familiar but still unsettling sight of their son hooked to innumerable IVs and tubes. Nick's little body lie there motionless, his chest covered in bandages, his arms taped down in an iron cross formation. They rubbed their son's head and legs, anywhere they were allowed to touch him. They sat by his bedside and held his little hands; they sat there for hours. The nurses seemed to be a constant presence in the room, always checking and adjusting equipment. They checked and rechecked Nick's vital signs, continuously monitoring all aspects of his recovery.

Not wanting to leave their child in the hospital alone, Tom and Chris stayed in one of the parent sleep rooms adjacent to the ICU. Tom and Chris shared one of the chairs that folded into a bed. They slept on the improvised bed, which was no wider than either one of their bodies, let alone both of their bodies. Every few hours one or both of them would rise to check on their son. They would visit in the earlier morning hours with nurses who worked the night shift in ICU, all the while watching Nick as he slowly made progress in his recovery.

Days after the surgery Nick was regaining consciousness, and was ready and able to breathe on his own. As the breathing tube was removed from Nick's throat and the ventilator was shut off, Nick began drawing in his first breaths after the surgery. Tom and Chris knew this was a tremendous leap in their son's recovery. Needing to get back to work, Tom left the hospital that evening. Chris, who hadn't left the hospital one time in all of her son's hospitalizations, remained in the ICU. She stayed at her son's side and continued to talk to him and read him stories. She continued to take short naps on the chair in one of the parent sleeping rooms. She would awaken several times a night and check on her son.

Everyday after work Tom would make the hour long drive into Minneapolis to Children's Hospital. He spent every evening with his wife in the ICU at Nick's side. Tom stayed late into the night before he left to drive an hour home, get settled into bed, and wake up a few hours later in order to go to work. On one of these evenings, Tom sat down at his son's bedside, thinking Nick looked peculiar.

"Chris, how come he is all puffy?" Tom asked while staring at his son.

Chris brushed his worries aside. "I have been here all day, and he doesn't look any different at all."

The nurse who had been working with Nick for nearly an entire shift agreed. "He looks the same, Tom. His ankles are not swollen, and his urine output has not decreased. He has not put on any extra fluid weight, either."

"No, look under his eyes, and look at his ears," Tom insisted. "He looks swollen."

Just then Nick coughed and his mouth opened wide. His tongue protruded from his mouth well past his lips. The swollen tongue blocked his airway and he began coughing, gagging, and choking. The next few minutes were a confusing blur for Tom and Chris as they were hurriedly pushed out of the way.

"We need a crash cart over here!" Nick's nurse hollered to the nearby nurses' station. A rush of commotion could be heard coming down the hall towards Nick's bed.

"Somebody page Anesthesia to the ICU, stat!" the charge nurse hollered as she came to Nick's side.

Tom and Chris held each other tight as they watched all of this play out in front of them from the corner of the room. Chris sobbed loudly, "I didn't notice! I didn't notice anything wrong with him!"

Tom tried to console her, but she continued. "He was fine! He was fine all day! I swear he was doing just fine!" A large crowd quickly formed around Nick's bed. Several doctors were trying to determine what had happened to their patient.

"Okay, his throat is swelling and we need to establish an airway!" the anesthesiologist ordered. "Intubate, and get ready to bag him." Nick's anesthesiologist began to slide the breathing tube into Nick's mouth and down his throat.

"Problem, it's not fitting!" the anesthesiologist yelled as she tried in vain to manipulate the tube.

"Smaller size!" the doctored barked. "Quickly, we don't have much time," he pleaded.

"His oxygen levels are dropping!" the charge nurse yelled.

Tom and Chris were absolutely powerless as they stood in the corner of the hospital room and watched their son's life seem to slip away right before their eyes.

"Yes! It's in!" Nick's nurse screamed.

"Good, bag him," the doctor said matter-of-factly. "Someone grab a ventilator. Let's get him stabilized."

Tom and Chris were still frozen in the corner of the room. Moments earlier they both were convinced they were watching their son die in front of them. Now, they stood there a second trying to understand the drama that played out in front of them.

The doctor approached them and said, "I don't know what happened. I will order some tests and hopefully we can determine if this was an allergic reaction, or something else." He walked over to the charge nurse, grabbed Nick's chart, and began writing.

Tom walked over to Nick, and looked down at his son. He was once again on the ventilator, not breathing on his own. Back to square one, Tom thought to himself as he held his son's hand.

"A leak. Air was leaking through a nick in his trachea, into the chest cavity," Dr. Stone told Tom and Chris. "During the surgery, when Nick was intubated, the breathing tube probably scraped along his trachea. The scrape allowed air to leak into the chest and be absorbed into the tissue. To treat Nick's air leak, we are going to be inserting and repositioning the chest tubes in order to drain the air out of Nick's chest. "The process will take several weeks."

Chris continued to stay by her son's side while the doctors worked to reduce the air trapped in Nick's body. He looked distorted and swollen; the excess air was absorbed into all of the soft tissue in his body. His ears, face, and scalp were stretched and bulging by the absorbed air. She hardly recognized her swollen baby. Several times a day the X-ray technicians would reposition Nick in order to take X-rays to determine where the floating pockets of air in his chest were located.

Each morning as Chris sat beside her son's side he would be X-rayed, and the new pocket of air would be identified in his chest. She held his hand and tried to comfort him while doctors inserted new drainage tubes into his chest to remove the excess air. Nick screamed as the doctor's cut into his chest to place the new tubes. He wrenched violently as they pulled the old tubes, which were several inches in length, out of him.

It pained her to watch Nick in such pain. Chris was there, no matter how painful it was to witness or how devastating it was to hear her child's screams; she stayed by his side. Nick's primary nurses cared for her and her needs as much as they cared for Nick. She leaned on them for support and they answered all her questions honestly.

Soon most of the excess air was drawn out of Nick's chest, and the days in which chest tubes needed to be moved became further and further apart. The swelling was decreasing all over his body. His face returned to normal, and he no longer looked like a monster. The doctors informed Nick's parents it was time to again remove the breathing tube, allowing him to breathe on his own.

Tom and Chris waited at Nick's bedside while Dr. Stone removed the breathing tube and disconnected the ventilator. Tom and Chris held each other while they watched Nick begin to draw in breaths on his own. Dr. Stone saw them waiting and holding each other and he said, "We won't know anything right away."

"When will we know? When do we know whether the nick in his trachea is healed?" Tom asked.

"We won't know anytime soon. We will monitor Nick to be sure no air is leaking," Dr. Stone said. For the next several days, Tom and Chris, along with Dr. Stone and many nurses, continued to monitor Nick's progress.

Days went by and there were no signs of air leaking into Nick's chest cavity, and tests were ordered every day to determine if small pockets of air were reforming. Nick made steady progress in his recovery and was soon ready to be discharged from the hospital.

Chris carried Nick out the front doors of the hospital; Tom was waiting next to the station wagon he had pulled up to the front door. Chris passed Nick to her husband and turned around to give the nurses, who had walked her outside, a hug.

"Thank you. Thank you for everything you have done for Nicholas," she said softly. "Thank you so much. I couldn't have done this without you."

Tom strapped Nick into his car seat and double-checked that everything was secure. He closed the left rear door to the station wagon, and walked over to his wife. He put his arm around her and said, "Well, are you ready to get out of here?"

Before they left, Tom also hugged the nurses one by one. "Thank you for taking care of Nick, and for being

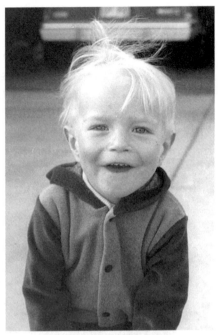

Nick 1983

there for Chris," he said. He choked up as he continued, "You will never know how comforting it was every night knowing you gals would be here watching over Nick, and helping Chris. I know I wouldn't have been able to continue working if you weren't here with my wife and my son. I am just so grateful you were there for us." It had been another six-week stay.

As time passed after Nicks second open heart surgery, Tom and Chris began to notice some remarkable changes. Although Nick's lips were still dark blue or purple in color and his fingernails were dark blue, he seemed to have more energy. He began moving around more on his own and became a more active child. When the neighborhood families would get together, Nick really enjoyed playing with the other children. While he still didn't have enough energy to keep pace with the other kids, Nick still loved the opportunity to be around them.

Tom and Chris also noticed that Nick's verbal skills really began to take off. All the time surrounded by doctors and nurses began to pay off as Nick began to soak up those interactions like a sponge. Just over three years old, he had a vocabulary well beyond his years. During trips to the supermarket people would stare as Nick (still quite small for a two-and-a-half-year-old) talked in full sentences to his parents. Chris also helped by reading to her son every night before he went to sleep. Nick oftentimes argued and tried to stay awake beyond his bedtime simply so he could have another story read to him.

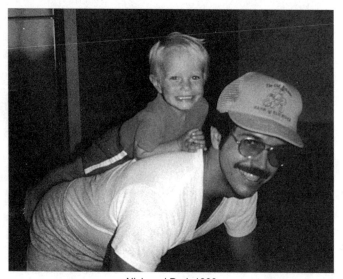

Nick and Dad, 1983

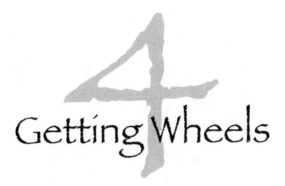

Getting Wheels

"So, what do you think?" I asked my mom.

"What? What do I think about what?" she asked.

"What do you think of my speech? You have read it about ten times now. Do you like it?" I asked, becoming confused.

"Yes, I do like it. I was just thinking about your graduation. I can't believe it is finally here," she said, smiling broadly.

"I know, the time has really flown by," I agreed.

I leaned back in my chair, and began thinking back to when I first started school. I remembered how hard I tried to keep up with the other kids, and most importantly fit in.

When I was about four years old, all of the other kids in my neighborhood began riding large plastic Big Wheel trikes around their yards, and back and forth to the children's homes. My best friend and next-door neighbor, Ryan Ebert, had the coolest Big Wheel, a black KIT Big Wheel modeled after the TV series Night Rider. I wanted a black Big Wheel like Ryan's in the worst way imaginable. I watched him all afternoon ride his Big Wheel around the driveway and I was so jealous. When I

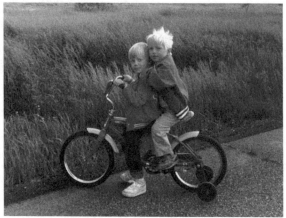

Nick and Ryan Ebert, 1985

went home in the afternoon I told my parents all about Ryan's new Big Wheel.

While my parents, my two older brothers, and I sat down for dinner, I could hardly contain how excited I was about Ryan's new toy. "Mom! Dad! Guess what Ryan got today!" I said loudly.

"Nick, shhh. We are right here," Mom replied.

Unphased by her lack of a guess I continued. "Ryan got the coolest new Big Wheel. It's a new Night Rider Big Wheel."

"Oh, wow," my dad said, feigning enthusiasm.

"Yeah, it's black with cool stickers, and it goes really fast." As I spoke about Ryan's new Big Wheel I became more and more excited. "It goes so fast; he was just going like this all over the driveway." I made an exaggerated zigzag motion with my hands while I was talking, just barely missing David's glass of milk.

"Nick, settle down and watch what you are doing," Mom scolded.

"It looks just like the one from the show," I continued, all but ignoring my mom's rebuke. "It is so cool, and, and I want one really bad!"

The dinner table was silent after my last comment; my brothers stared down at their plates. Mom watched Dad chew his food intently. My dad finished chewing his food, swallowed hard, and took a long drink of his milk. He sat down his glass of milk, looked across the table at me, and momentarily crushed my dreams.

"Nick, you know you don't have enough energy to peddle yourself around on a Big Wheel. You won't be able to do it," he said calmly. My face dropped and I put my head in my hands.

"Listen, your mother and I want you to be happy, but we also need you to stay healthy. If you get one of those and try to peddle it around and keep up with Ryan and your other friends, you will just get more worn down."

Tears fell from my face onto my plate of mashed potatoes. I was embarrassed and tried to secretly wipe off my face and clear my throat. I tried desperately to hold off the growing wave of emotion, but I was unable to contain it. As I began to cry harder I looked up at my parents and yelled, "I don't care! I don't want to be sick. I just want to play with my friends!" I then stood up abruptly and ran to the bedroom where I curled up with my stuffed animals on my bed and cried myself to sleep.

Of course my parents were right, I couldn't have peddled a Big Wheel around our street. At that point I could hardly walk one house next door to play with Ryan. Once I did walk over, I either played there for several hours until I felt like I could make it home, or until Ryan's older brother Chad carried me home on his back. But, none of that mattered or made sense then; the only thing I cared about was having a Big Wheel just like Ryan.

Like most children, I didn't have the will power to stay mad at my parents for any length of time. I still loved them and admired them, even though they hadn't given me what I had wanted. In the weeks following, my mom must have told my godparents Aunt Germaine, Uncle Bob and Uncle Eugene, how upset I was that I couldn't keep up with my friends by riding a big wheel. A few months later, at Christmas, I received quite a surprising gift from them.

"Nick, come out into the garage for a second!" Uncle Eugene yelled after all the other gifts had been opened. I began walking down the stairs from the family room of my aunt and uncle's house, wondering why people were gathered around the garage door. I walked into the entryway and dug around in the closet for boots. I slid on my boots, and was just about to open the door leading to the garage when Uncle Eugene, Aunt Germaine, and Uncle Bob all came inside from the garage and said, "Nick! Come out here!"

I followed my parents into the garage, and noticed the entire family huddled into the garage. In the center of the garage I saw the most amazing thing waiting for me. "What is that?" I asked.

"Well, Nick, THAT is better then a Big Wheel!" Uncle Eugene replied, obviously very excited.

I could not believe my eyes. Sitting in the garage was a battery-powered, go-cart style car, the kind I had only seen a few times on television commercials. It was a Power Wheels car, and I was absolutely shocked.

"We want you to be able to play with your friends, Nick, and this way you will be able to keep up with them," Aunt Germaine explained.

Just then Uncle Bob reached into the small plastic car and powered up the car. He explained all of the controls, and showed me what to do to make it go as fast as possible. I was jumping up and down anxiously awaiting to drive it. Soon I was able to climb into the car and drive around the garage while my family watched.

My parents were standing in the corner of the garage with their arms around each other. My mom kept telling my godparents that this was too much, and that they didn't have

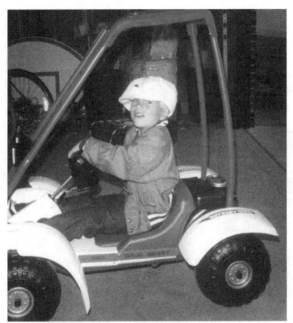

Nick in his *Baja Beast* electric car, given to him by his
godparents, 1986

to do that for me. My parents wrapped their arms around my
godparents and thanked them for their kindness.

I drove my little battery-powered car everywhere. I loved
to get out of my car wearing my father's altered police uniform
and walk up to him with notepad in hand. We played cops and
robbers, and now I had my very own police car. When Ryan and
the other neighborhood kids peddled their Big Wheels down
the street, I would ride along with them, and then easily pass
them and laugh. For the first time in my life, not only was I
able to keep up with other kids, but I could beat them. For the
first time in my life, kids I knew had a reason to be envious
of me.

When I started kindergarten I was more excited than most
kids. I was so excited to be able to go to school like my older
brothers. Going to kindergarten also meant I was going to meet
new friends, something I was really looking forward to.

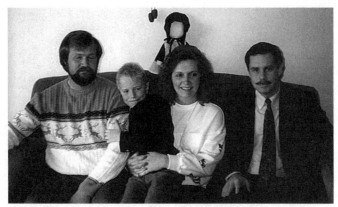

All of Nick's godparents. From left to right: Uncle Eugene Zerwas,
Nick, Aunt Germaine and Uncle Bob Yochum, 1986.

"Nick, hurry up, you don't want to be last on your first day," my mom yelled from the kitchen in our house. She was just finishing up talking with a local newspaper reporter, Stephanie Klinzing, who had asked to write a story about my first day of school. I walked down the stairs into the kitchen, smiling broadly, showing off my freshly combed hair and my new clothes. My dad followed closely behind, ushering me towards the door and out to the end of the driveway to wait for the bus.

The newspaper reporter took a few photos while I walked to the end of the driveway. My brothers were already at the end of the driveway waiting for the bus, along with some other kids in the neighborhood. As I boarded the bus and found a place to sit, my brothers watched at a distance to ensure that everything went smoothly. I sat in my seat, looking around in amazement at all the other kids already on the bus. Kids were laughing and yelling, telling the stories of their summer vacation away from school. I was amazed at the amount of energy these kids had. They seemed to be almost lifting right out of their seats.

As the bus pulled into the school I hesitated slightly, but soon got the cue from my brothers and followed them off of the school bus. My kindergarten teacher, Ms. Ostroot, was waiting on the sidewalk, watching students get off their buses. Standing next to her was the same newspaper reporter who was taking my picture at my house. She snapped a few more photos of me and then followed me into the building. I followed Ms. Ostroot into the school all the way into the classroom. A large group of very uncertain kindergarten students was already forming. Students were milling about looking at the posters hanging on the walls. Some of the kids recognized a few other children from other activities, but most were like me and didn't know anybody. I sat down in the corner of the classroom and began playing with a few Legos that were already lying out on the floor. While I sat on the ground the other children ran around and played tag, or just hustled and bustled throughout the room. I had been in kindergarten for about fifteen minutes watching the other students run around, and I was already exhausted.

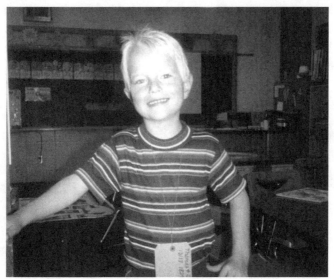

Nick on his first day of kindergarten

Watching all of these other children laugh, yell, and run around was the first time I really understood how much different I was from the normal kids. I watched them from the corner of the room as they ran around making new friends, and I was jealous. I was able to talk and play with the kids near me, and eventually I made several good friendships, but I will never forget that first day of kindergarten in the corner of the room.

One of the things I liked most about being in kindergarten was answering questions. I loved raising my hand, and saying a correct answer in front of the class. There was nothing better than everyone in class seeing how good I was at school. I couldn't play as hard as them and I wasn't as strong, but I felt like I was much smarter then they were. Feeling smart gave me self-confidence to talk to the other kids and try to make new friends. I didn't worry about what people thought about my pale complexion or blue lips and fingers, because I was a really good student.

Kindergarten went by quickly for both my parents and me. As the year went on I became more comfortable being around other kids. Soon I was no longer jealous of the kids who were bigger than me and had more energy than I did. After a while

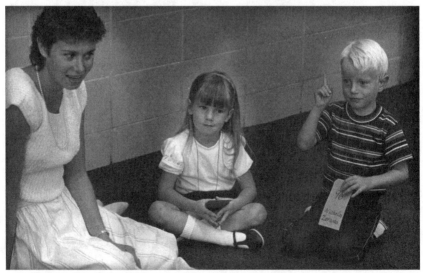

Teacher Tina Ostroot, left, watches as Nick answers a question in kindergarten.

my parents became more comfortable with me being gone for half of the day.

As time passed and I crept ever closer to seven years old, my parents and I would meet with Dr. Stone. My doctor's appointments were every few months, and I could tell my parents were always nervous and upset beforehand, and a little calmer afterwards. As time passed it was becoming evident to nearly everyone but me that I was not doing as well as I had been. My parents noticed less frequent trips up the stairs to my bedroom, and a few extra pounds of water weight. Dr. Stone noticed a drop in my cardiac output, low perfusion, and decreased exercise tolerance. Once in a while I noticed an upset tummy.

My parents and Dr. Stone were very aware that as I was getting older my body was demanding more oxygen—oxygen my struggling heart was simply unable to provide. In talking with Dr. Stone my parents always held out hope for a miracle. Dr. Stone, however, tried to keep their hopes in check, and reminded them their son was very sick and didn't have long to live.

A few months before I turned seven years old I started first grade at Handke Elementary School. This was my first time in a real, full-time school. I was very excited because this would be the year students would begin to read, and I was already an excellent reader. My first grade class was almost entirely new kids; I didn't know anyone from my kindergarten class the year before. On the first day of class I was once again taken back by the energy level of the students in my class. As I sat in my desk and watched the other kids race around the room, I was really in awe of what they could do. They would laugh and run around a few desks, and then stand there and talk some more without looking the slightest bit fatigued. I was finding it difficult to remain standing for more than a few minutes, and it was nearly impossible to walk any long distances without feeling sick to my stomach.

I would follow the other children outside to recess and watch as they ran around and played different games, like cops and robbers and tag. I would sit on the railroad ties that bordered the large sand pit that surrounded the jungle gym. As the other kids would pass the time playing touch football or kickball, I would visit with recess monitors.

Sometimes as students were filtering inside from recess and lunch I would go straight back to class and talk with my first grade teacher. When I talked to Mrs. Fournier, I told her things I would never say to my mom. I would climb into her lap and tell her about being sick. I would explain that I didn't like how I was starting to feel, and that it was no fun having a sick heart. At seven years old I even told Mrs. Fournier that I was afraid I was going to die, and that made me sad for my brothers and for my mom and dad. This poor woman would hold me in her arms and cry and tell me everything was going to be okay, and not to worry about my family. She spent countless lunches with a first grader on her lap telling her he was going to die soon. Mrs. Fournier was always there, she listened every time I wanted to talk. This first grade teacher doubled as a psychologist.

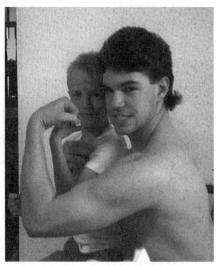
Nick and Tommy, 1987

A Wish
For The Fontan

As I rode down to Children's Hospital in Minneapolis, I could tell my mom and dad were more anxious than usual. Dr. Stone met us as we walked into the waiting room of the clinic. He reached down and picked me up and said, "Come back with me, big guy." My parents followed Dr. Stone as he carried me back towards the exam rooms. He veered right and dropped me off with the X-ray technician, asking my parents to follow him back to the exam room.

"Well," Dr. Stone began with a bright look in his eyes, "I think there is something we can try for Nicholas. There is a new surgical procedure that Nick may be a candidate for."

"Procedure! What kind of procedure?" my mom immediately asked.

"Well, it is a surgery that would reroute the blood through Nick's heart and change how his heart delivers blood throughout his body." Dr. Stone slowly began to explain. "We would change how Nick's heart pumps so that his left side would only pump blood to his body, like in normal hearts. His right atrium would do the work for the entire right side of the heart and pump blood to the lungs."

My dad jumped in, "How is that better? Why not let the stronger left ventricle keep pumping instead of the right atrium?"

"Well, by separating the two sides of the heart, the blood with oxygen won't mix with the blood without oxygen. This will allow the heart to work more efficiently," Dr. Stone explained.

My mom, obviously excited, rattled off several questions. "Has this been done before? Who would do the surgery? Is it experimental? How risky is it?"

"Okay, let me try to answer those questions one at a time," Dr. Stone began. "This surgery is called the Fontan procedure; it is named after Dr. Fontan who first performed it. This surgery has been attempted once before in Minnesota on a little girl from Duluth...her surgery was unsuccessful. The surgery is very risky, but we feel that it is the only option for Nick. Without surgical intervention Nick will not be able to maintain this minimum level of cardiac output for any length of time," Dr. Stone explained with a look of grave concern on his face.

"Odds? What kind of odds do we have with a surgery like this?" my dad stammered. "I mean, is it fifty-fifty, or sixty-forty? What are the chances that this will actually work?"

"Well, it is a new surgery, and it is very risky. If you do decide to do the Fontan procedure the chances of survival for Nick would not be greater then twenty-eighty," he said as he looked across the table at my parents.

"Eighty percent—those are good odds..." my mom started.

"No," Dr. Stone quickly interrupted, "twenty-eighty; twenty percent chance he will survive and an eighty percent chance that he will not." There was a hint of pain in his voice.

"Oh...ummm...Oh, I see," was all that my mom could say.

"What if we do nothing, what if we don't have the surgery and we just wait and see what happens? What are the odds for Nick then?" my dad asked.

"If we wait and do nothing, the chances of Nick surviving without the surgery are zero. He will not live another year if you don't do the Fontan'" Dr. Stone quietly explained.

My parents looked at each other and knew they were both together, and felt they had to give me every opportunity in the world to succeed. They squeezed each other's hands and looked at Dr. Stone and nodded their heads. I would have the Fontan surgery.

As news of my impending heart surgery spread around town, several people approached my parents wanting to know how to help. Friends and family prepared meals and watched my older bothers. The Elk River Jaycees, a local charity organization, spearheaded a fundraising drive. The Jaycee's raised enough money to send my entire family to Orlando, Florida, to visit Walt Disney World a few weeks before my surgery.

Our trip to Disney World was unbelievable. I was unable to walk for any distance at this point, but my parents pushed me around in a wheelchair, and I was able to go on most of the rides. My dad let me go on Magic Mountain—over my mom's protest. This vacation was unforgettable for my family, a week where we were able to forget about surgery, forget about only living to be seven years old, and a time to focus on having fun together as a family.

One of the last days before we left Disney World I asked my dad for some change for the wishing well. He pulled a penny out of his pocket and tried to give it to me. I told him I had a pretty big wish, so I was going to need a quarter. He chuckled to himself, reached back into his pocket, and pulled out a quarter. I took that quarter, held it in my hand for a while, and then threw it into the fountain.

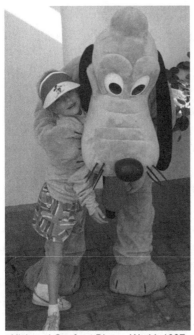

Nick and Goofy at Disney World, 1987

Later that afternoon when my dad asked what I had wished for, I turned and said, "To feel better; all I want is to feel healthy."

My dad rubbed my back and hugged me, and as he held me next to him he said, "I know, Bud, that's all any of us want right now."

The following day we flew back to Minnesota and began preparing for my surgery. The night before the surgery I was admitted into Children's Hospital for observation and some pre-op blood tests. I had a hospital room with a single bed on the seventh floor. As evening set in, the people I was very close with began coming to my hospital room to wish me luck for tomorrow. My grandparents on both sides of the family, along with my great grandma Zerwas, came to the hospital to wish me luck. Neighbors, friends, aunts, uncles, and cousins all made the trip down to the hospital to see me the night before the surgery. I sat on my hospital bed and visited with three of my cousins while the room continued to fill with well wishers. As I looked over my cousin Matt's shoulder and across the room, I realized the room was full of people, and even more people were standing in the hallway outside of my room waiting to come in and say hi.

As people filed past me to say hi and wish me good luck, a few cried while they were talking to me, and most looked like they had been crying. I grabbed a hold of the people as they filtered by, and thanked them for coming and for praying for me. I cracked jokes endlessly in an attempt to lift the rather sullen mood. I told funny stories about people as I saw them make their way through the door into my room. I did whatever I could to change the subject off of my surgery. Looking back at that night, it reminds me of people filing past a casket at a wake, except I wasn't dead yet.

As the last visitors left it was already well past my usual bedtime. I should have been exhausted, but I knew I wouldn't be able to sleep. My mom made her bed in the foldout chair in the corner of my room, and then tucked me into bed. I lay there as she turned out the lights, and continued to stare at the ceiling. I didn't dare close my eyes for fear that I would fall asleep, only to wake up just in time for the surgery. While I lay in bed I thought a lot about what Dr. Stone had said about this surgery, not about the risks or the odds. I thought instead about how much better I was going to feel after the surgery, and what it would be like to no longer have purple lips and blue fingernails. As I finally fell asleep that night, I dreamed that I was walking in a park. I walked all around and played with the other kids and laughed and joked. In my dream I was able to keep up with them. And nobody said anything about how I looked, because I looked just like them, with pink lips and fingernails. In my dream I was so happy to be feeling that wonderful.

"Nick. Nick, honey, time to get up," my mom quietly whispered to me. I rolled over and opened my eyes, straining to make out her image in the still dark room. I looked around, momentarily forgetting I had spent the night in the hospital. As I rolled my body, my hand with the IV in it bumped the side guardrail of my bed. The slight twinge of pain jolted me out of my sleepy state. I sat up in bed rubbing my hand while my mom continued to talk.

"Nick, time to get up, you have a big day," she said encouragingly. She was already completely dressed in fresh clothes and was folding up the reclining chair she had spent the night on.

Moments later my dad walked into the room carrying two large coffees from McDonald's and a bag of egg and cheese McMuffins. He passed a coffee to my mom, and sat down in the reclining chair. He offered me an egg McMuffin and my mom abruptly swatted at his hand.

"He can't eat anything," she said sharply.

"Oh, yeah…oops," he replied with a sheepish smile on his face.

"Don't worry, I am not that hungry this morning anyway," I said to my dad. "I just wish we could get the show on the road."

"I know, Bud, soon enough," he replied as he reached over and squeezed my foot.

A while later my nurse came into the room and began preparing things for me to go downstairs to pre-op. She gave me a little Dixie cup with purple liquid and told me it was like grape Kool-Aid, but I nearly threw up. As I lay in the bed she started switching all of the IV pumps and heart monitors onto stands that would roll along with the bed. Before long the nurse had me moving out of my hospital room and headed downstairs into the pre-op unit.

As we arrived in my private pre-op room I was already starting to become very sleepy. The purple Kool-Aid the nurse had given me upstairs was really kicking in. My Grandma Helga came in the pre-op room and brought along with her my two older brothers, David and Tom. The three of them all looked very tired. David and Tom looked as though they had just gotten done crying. Their faces were red and their eyes were swollen and blood shot. They were both clearing their throats and sniffing loudly as they came into my room.

"Tommy! David!" I shouted with a smile. "I am so glad you guys made it," I said with a smile. I sat up in bed and extended my arms out for a hug from both of them. As they hugged me Tom replied, "Well, of course we made it."

"That's great," I continued in a loud voice. "I am just so glad to have the whole family together." Tom and David both sat down on the edge of my bed. My parents closed in behind them, creating a very tight circle around my bed.

"Nick," my mom started off, "we are all praying so hard that everything works out..." As her words trailed off into tears, my father jumped in almost on cue.

"Bud," he started off, "if anyone can do this I know you can. You are going to fight. Just keep fighting...just keep fighting," he pleaded with me.

"We...we believe in you, Nick...and...we know you can do this...and we love you so...much," David managed, though just a few words came in between sobs.

My brother Tom just hugged me and cried—he couldn't get a single word out. He just squeezed me tightly and cried loudly into my ear. He stayed like that until my dad finally peeled him off of me.

My parents composed themselves as the anesthesiologist came into the room. The doctor and my parents discussed the risks surrounding putting me to sleep for the surgery. I listened just enough to ensure that I wouldn't be awake for the operation. As the doctor finished explaining the procedure one last time, a nurse entered the room and began unlocking the wheel brakes on my bed.

Realizing they were about to roll me out of the pre-op room and into surgery, I smiled and waved good-bye to my parents and my brothers. Tom and David leaned over and began hugging me tightly and crying very hard. My parents placed their hands on the shoulders of Tom and David and gently pulled them back. As I was being wheeled towards the door I watched my family cling to each other, barely being able to stand. I sat up in bed slightly, and in my highly sedated state I calmly said, "Hey, don't act so sad—the surgery will only last a few hours. I will see you this evening." With that I lay my head down and fell asleep.

After the surgery I was wheeled out of the OR into the Intensive Care Unit while I was still out from the anesthesia. My parents were allowed into the ICU while I began to come around. My small hospital room was filled with nurses monitoring and changing IV pumps and medications. Dr. Stone spent the first few hours after surgery at a small desk in the entry to my room, keeping watch over every detail. My parents were relegated to a small area near the head of my bed, where they could stand without blocking the nurses from reaching one of the monitors or machines helping to keep me alive.

As I began to wake up I was immediately preoccupied with the pain in my throat. My parents talked repeatedly about how well I was recovering and how great the surgery went, but all I could focus on was my sore throat. The breathing tube in my throat was causing the discomfort. The large tube allowed my body to be supplied with oxygen, but made it impossible for me to speak and was the cause of the irritation and pain in my throat. As I began to awaken I fought against the respirator and coughed violently. My parents did their best to console and calm me as best they could. As I became more coherent I was able to relax and adjust to the respirator tube and listen more intensively to the people around me.

When I was able to stay awake for more than just a few minutes at a time, my nurses brought something to my bedside to show me. A small crowd of doctors, nurses and family gathered as the nurses held the object in front of my face for me to see. I strained to focus straight ahead, and I realized I was staring into a small hand mirror. After a few seconds of staring into the mirror I noticed what everyone had been trying to tell me earlier. I looked at my face in the mirror, and for the first time I was seeing what I had always hoped for—I was looking at the face of a normal child. My lips were no longer dark purple, and my face was no longer ashen gray. I finally had pink lips and bright rosy cheeks! My face strained as I struggled to control my body and raise my right hand. My dad, understanding what I was trying to do, helped guide my hand in front of my face. I looked at my fingers and began to cry harder when I saw pink fingernails. That's when I realized the surgery actually did work, and everything was going to be okay.

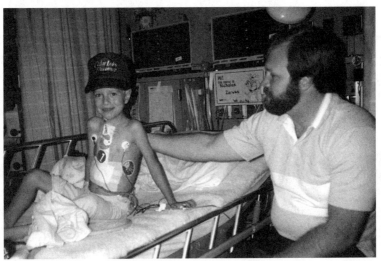

Nick and Uncle Eugene after third surgery, 1987

The following day I was relieved to find out the breathing tube was going to be pulled, and I was finally going to be able to have something to drink. When the anesthesiologist came into my room, he explained the steps to removing the breathing tube and told me the sore throat would last a few days. With that, he pulled some of the tape off my face and began ordering me to breathe in and out. The third time he ordered me to exhale he pulled with one quick motion, and I could feel the breathing tube rising out of my body. I coughed and gagged after it was finally out, but I was relieved to be able to fully swallow, and I was looking forward to some Kool-Aid.

"Wow, I am so glad to have that thing out!" I told my parents. My parents both turned their heads and looked at me.

"What did you say?" my mom asked.

"I said, I am so glad to have the breathing tube out." As I talked I noticed it took me a while to manage to get the words out; I was interrupted several times mid sentence as I ran out of breath. My parents looked at each other, and my dad said something softly to my mom, but I was unable to make it out. I was not too concerned with them; my mind was preoccupied by the need to have something to drink. My nurse would not allow me to have a glass of juice right away; instead, she gave my mom a small cup with some ice chips for me to start with. Mom would scoop a few ice chips into the spoon and place them carefully on my tongue. I savored the cool ice as it melted on my tongue and made its way down my sore throat.

Throughout the day I chewed on ice chips, and eventually sipped on rationed amounts of fruit punch. My throat began to feel better, and I was no longer burdened with the need to soothe my throat. I instead began to more fully notice that every time I began to speak my soft voice would run out of air. I could not complete a sentence without stopping for air. I could tell my parents believed something was wrong as well, because my mom began talking with nurses, and a few doctors I didn't recognize had come in to my room to see me. The new doctors asked me a few questions, and then looked in my mouth and asked me to make vowel sounds.

Soon Dr. Stone came into my hospital room and sat down. Dr. Stone looked around the room at my parents and me, cleared his throat and began. "Well, we have looked into Nick's speech problem, and have evaluated the function of his vocal chords. It does appear as though one of his vocal chords is paralyzed, and that appears to be causing his decreased volume and increased pitch. It would also explain the choppy speech pattern, as he needs to stop frequently in order to inhale another breath."

"Paralyzed?" my dad began. "Is that going to be permanent? I mean, will his regular voice ever come back?"

"We don't know yet, Tom," Dr. Stone replied. "We won't be able to tell for quite a while. There does seem to be nerve damage done. However, the extent of that damage is unknown."

"Okay, well when will we know for sure? Will it just come back in a month, six months, a year, or five years?" my dad asked.

"Probably longer than a month, but if it's going to come back, it would do so in less than a year," Dr. Stone explained.

"But, you don't think that will happen," my mom offered.

"Chris, I wouldn't say that. I don't know if it will come back. It might come back, or it might not, but I just don't know." Dr. Stone continued with a look of understanding. "Listen, I know we didn't bargain for this, but this is minor considering what could have happened."

"Who cares! I am alive," I said. "If someone doesn't like me because of my voice, they wouldn't have been a good friend anyway. The surgery worked, and that's all that matters."

"Bud, you're right. We just wanted to understand what happened," Dad told me as he patted my leg and smiled.

We thanked Dr. Stone for explaining everything to us, and for all of his help with everything. My mom hugged him and my dad shook his hand, and they again commended him on all of his hard work and for helping me through this.

Before Dr. Stone left, he told me I would have my chest tubes removed the following day and I would be able to leave the Intensive Care Unit.

The next morning a surgeon from Dr. Nicoloff's group came into my room to remove my three chest tubes. I was sitting up in bed watching some cartoons when he came through the door. My nurse followed closely behind, and was already uncapping a syringe and drawing up some drugs. At first I didn't realize why she seemed to be in such a hurry. Then I noticed the surgeon was already at my bedside removing the

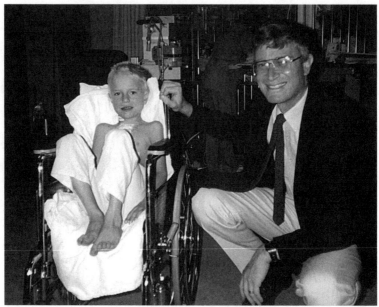
Nick and Dr. Stone after third surgery, 1987

bandages surrounding my chest tubes. While the surgeon pulled at the tape on my stomach, my nurse injected the syringe into the IV in my forearm.

"Okay, Nick, it's time to pull out those tubes," the doctor said without looking up from his work.

"Doctor, I just gave the narcotics; it hasn't had enough time to work yet," the nurse told him in an urgent voice.

"Well, it will be quick enough," he replied. He looked up and said with a smile, "It will be over before you even know I've started."

Knowing full well whatever was about to happen was going to hurt very badly, I began to breathe very rapidly. I looked across the room at my mom who was already moving towards my bedside. She sat next to me and rubbed my arm while she held my hand.

The doctor gave me a disapproving look and asked, "Why are you crying? I haven't even done anything yet." He finished removing the rest of the bandages and then laid out a green towel across my stomach. "Okay!" the doctor said loudly, with an obviously fake enthusiasm. "I am going to count to three. On three I want you to breathe out and just keep breathing out as much as you can."

"Uh…okay," I stammered through my breaths as I looked around the room frantically, trying to find someone to help me.

"One!" the doctor said very loudly.

"Uh… I…uh…" My mind raced as I tried to find something to say to make him stop.

"Two!" he continued.

"Umm…Wai…" I begged, hoping for more time.

"Three!" he said, cutting me off mid plea as he jerked his arm backward removing the six inches of tubing that was inside my abdomen.

"Ahhhhh! Ohhhh!" I screamed as I felt the tubing twist and wind throughout my body, convinced several of my organs also came out with the chest tubes. I instantly felt nauseous. My uneasiness was not helped when I looked down at the bloody tubes lying on the cloth draped across my lap. I panted and hyperventilated as I tried to regain my breath.

The doctor looked up, patted me on the head and said, "See, now, that wasn't too bad."

I looked across the bed at him through my tears in disbelief. I continued crying and coughing and tried with all my strength not to vomit. A few moments after he left, the drugs the nurse had given to me earlier put me quickly to sleep.

The next morning I was transferred out of the ICU to finish my hospital stay. Exactly one week after my surgery I was released from Minneapolis Children's Hospital. Dr. Stone checked in on me that morning, and he and my parents talked about how amazed they all were with my quick recovery. I gave Dr. Stone a hug as I thanked him for everything. Two of my nurses walked with my parents as they wheeled me to the lobby of the hospital. We thanked them for all they had done, and everyone cried as I climbed into the back seat of my parent's station wagon. As I turned and waved to my nurses, I felt like I was leaving part of my family behind.

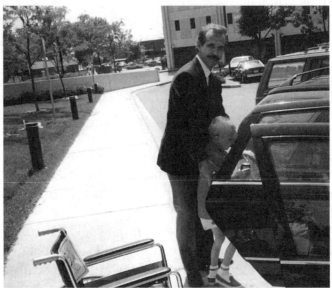

Nick and Dad leaving Children's Hospital after third surgery, 1987

The "Sick Freak"

I recovered from the surgery very quickly at home. Each day I had a little bit more energy, and I was able to do more and more things. Soon, I was able to walk distances that I was unable to walk in the months leading up to the surgery. Stairs were no longer a struggle to climb, and I was able to remain active for an entire day without feeling ill.

My raspy voice never bothered me, and, in fact, I hardly even noticed it at first. I only realized the difference when I was talking to people, and I had to keep pausing mid sentence to take breaths. I also noticed that I wasn't able to talk as loud as I could before, and so sometimes people had trouble hearing me.

Other people noticed my voice, and they immediately recognized something was different about me. When ever I met other kids for the first time, they would make a face or giggle when I started talking, assuming I was joking around. Adults would look at me and ask, "Are you okay?" Or, "Are you losing your voice?" Every time I met somebody new, I was forced to explain during the first few minutes of the conversation about my heart problem, my surgeries, and my damaged vocal chord.

Someone always seemed to ask, "Are you catching a cold?" Or the ever popular, "Oh man, what's wrong with your voice?"

That fall when I started back to school, I really struggled with playing with other kids and making new friends. I still didn't have as much energy as everybody else, even though I was feeling much better than I had the year prior. I still couldn't run around on the playground with my friends, though, and if I talked to new people at school they wanted to know why I was talking funny.

In elementary school my self-esteem was pretty low. I knew and fully understood that it was by the grace of God, and a total miracle, that I was even alive. However, I truly believed I wasn't as good as the other kids at my school. I felt like a sick freak, and I just knew that I did not belong. Watching the other kids play together, I understood that I did not fit and that I never would fit in. Some kids in my school constantly mocked and teased me for running like a girl and talking like a girl. Those kids constantly mocked my voice, and degraded me in front of as many other students as they could. On those days I would come home absolutely crushed and cry at the kitchen table.

As I would cry to my mom, and tell her about what the kids said or did to me that day, I would get upset and demand to know why I wasn't like everyone else. On one of those occasions my mom sat me down, and explained a whole new way to look at myself. In the course of this one conversation my mom affected the entire way I have approached my life. She looked right at me and said, "Nick, God has a plan for everyone he puts on Earth, and everyone he puts on Earth has a special gift to bring to the world. God only gives each person as much difficulty in their life as they can handle, and God knows you can deal with everything you have had to deal with. You do have a gift from God, a special talent. But don't be upset, Nick, that your talent isn't running fast or playing professional sports. God gave you the gift of brains. You are so smart at math and at science, and you are such a good reader. Your gift from God will allow you to go through college and change the world."

I was crying hard as I listened to mom tell me about the positive things in my life. I very much identified with being a survivor, and so to hear her talk about that was very rewarding. After she finished her pep talk I gave her a big hug and thanked her for cheering me up. Before I went upstairs to my bedroom to read I asked my mom one last question. "Mom, if God gives everyone one special gift, then what's your special gift from God?"

My mom stared at me blankly for a second and then replied, "Well, Nick, it takes some people a little longer in life to figure that out."

I smiled back at my mom and reassured her, "I bet it is your chocolate chip cookies." With that I went upstairs to my room to read.

From that day on I never again watched the other children enviously as they ran around the playground. I began to focus on schoolwork and grades, and learning the most from class everyday I was there. The kids who had been mean to me now left me alone when they realized I would no longer give the upset reaction they were looking for when they teased someone.

I enjoyed going to school and meeting new people once I was no longer concerned about what every person I met was going to think of me. I developed an attitude where if someone wanted to be nice to me and be my friend, that was great, but if they didn't want to, I wasn't upset by that either. I figured out early on that I couldn't make people like me, and I couldn't force other kids to by my friends. I also understood early on that not everyone would understand me, and not every kid would want to be my friend. That understanding really helped me deal with the pressures of kids being mean to me and teasing me all throughout grade school.

By the time I was in sixth grade the people in my elementary school knew me well enough to understand my physical limitations, and my unique approach to friendships. What nobody realized that year was that my health was declining quickly.

Early in the school year, I was heading inside from recess, coming from the Handke Pit, a sunken stadium behind the school. The Pit, as it was called, was well below street level and served as the stadium for the old high school. Large flights of stairs flanked both sides of the pit, and served as the only entrances and exits. After recess, while I was climbing the stairs out of the pit to return to the school, I began to feel weak and tired. Those feelings persisted with me, and developed into a nausea that stuck with me for the rest of the day. Nervous about not feeling well after climbing the stairs, I monitored what activities I was able to do very closely over the next few days.

During those days I noticed I was unable to stand for long periods of time, and I realized the afternoon naps I had been taking after school might be a sign of something more serious. After I was totally convinced that something might be going on with my heart I decided it was time to talk to my parents. We were seated at the dinner table, and my dad just finished telling us a story from work. I had remained nearly silent during supper until I gathered the courage needed to ruin dinner, and devastate my parents.

"Mom, Dad, I...I think there is something wrong," I said quietly across the dinner table. I was unable to complete my first sentence without beginning to cry. My parents stopped eating, turned their heads, and stared at me. "I don't feel well. I don't feel well," I kept repeating to them.

"What do you mean?" my dad asked, as his voice slightly rose.

"I mean that I can't do what I used to be able to do. When I try doing those things I feel sick." I began to cry harder, but

I tried to keep eating, hoping if I focused on my food I could make the tears go away.

"Things...what things?" my dad demanded.

"Feel sick? What do you mean, feel sick?" my mom asked, looking confused.

"I don't know...things. When I went up the stairs the other day at the Pit, I felt like I was going to puke for the rest of the day. And everyday when I get home from school I am so exhausted I fall asleep." As I spoke, I felt like I was presenting a case with evidence and exhibits to a jury. "By sick, I mean I am tired if I walk a lot, or stand a lot. I feel sick to my stomach and short of breath," I continued, stating my case.

"Short of breath!" my dad interrupted me. "Well, why did you wait so long to say something?" I could tell he was being overloaded with information. "How long have you been feeling tired and sick to your stomach?" he continued.

"I don't know. I have been tired for a few weeks, but feeling sick to my stomach just started a couple of days ago." I struggled to get the words out, and I was now crying heavily.

"Well, I will call Dr. Stone in the morning, and maybe he can get you in tomorrow afternoon," my mom said. Her face was flush, but she did her best to remain calm in front of me.

"One day at a time," my dad said softly, after having recovered from the initial shock of the news. "That's all you can do, Nick, is take it one day at a time. That's all any of us can do."

The next morning my mom called the heart clinic and Dr. Stone made time in his day for us, just like he did any time we needed to see him. After we arrived, Dr. Stone listened to me describe the feelings in my stomach, along with how climbing stairs or how walking a lot would bring on those feelings. He sat next to me and listened as I told him about not having enough energy to get through the day, and needing to take naps in the afternoon.

After listening for nearly fifteen minutes, Dr. Stone looked up at my parents and said, "Well, Nick, if you say you aren't feeling well, then I think we need to run a few tests and see if we can figure out what is going on."

With that he scheduled a follow-up appointment to run a stress test, where I would walk on a treadmill while my heart was being monitored. There would also be a heart catheterization, in which a balloon would travel up a blood vessel and into my heart in order to take measurements.

I went back to class after my appointment with Dr. Stone, but I had a hard time concentrating on school. I was consumed by tracking the things throughout the day that made me feel sick, and comparing to that to what I could do a few months earlier. Shortly after noticing the drop in my activity level my sixth grade teacher, Mr. Stensgard, asked if I would talk with him after class.

"Nick, I have noticed you seem more preoccupied lately," he began. "You seem a little withdrawn from the class. Is everything all right?"

As he spoke I could feel my face get warm, and thoughts of how to change the subject raced through my mind. I looked up at him, pleading with him to stop, but he continued.

"I don't know, Nick, but it just seems like you aren't having fun. Are you feeling okay?" he asked matter-of-factly.

I began to cry. Before I even realized it the tears were running down my cheeks, and I was sobbing into my hands. I tried to stop the tears, I coughed to clear my throat, but the tears kept coming, and soon I stopped trying to fight them. Mr. Stensgard looked down with a stunned look on his face as he watched me breakdown in front of him. I noticed his look of uneasiness, and I immediately felt bad for putting him in this position. I wiped the tears from my eyes and regained my composure. I sat down in my desk, and began talking to him.

"Mr. Stensgard, I am sorry for crying like that. It's just that I…"

"No, Nick, don't be sorry. You don't need to apologize," he said, his voice full of empathy.

"It's just that I haven't been feeling well lately, and I don't know what's happening. I went to see Dr. Stone, my cardiologist, and he has scheduled some more tests. I am trying not to think about it until I know something, but it's hard sometimes. Just walking around I can tell I can't do things that I was able to do before." I spoke fast, unloading on Mr. Stensgard.

"What things can't you do?" he asked. "I haven't noticed you not doing things."

"Well, I can still do most things, but when I do things like walk too much, or go up a bunch of stairs, I feel sick to my stomach and out of breath," I explained.

"Oh, I guess I haven't really noticed anything like that," he said.

"Yeah, neither did my parents. I really didn't pick up on it until a little over a month ago. But now I notice it everyday. Everyday when I come back from recess I feel all worn out and sick to my stomach. That's just from walking out there after lunch, standing around outside, and then walking back inside to class."

"Nick, is there anything I can do? I mean, what can I do to help you out?" Mr. Stensgard asked.

"I don't really think so, Mr. Stensgard. I don't know what you could do to keep me from feeling all worn out," I said.

"Would it help if you didn't have to go to recess? What if you stayed inside? That would cut down on your walking, and maybe you wouldn't feel as sick," Mr. Stensgard suggested.

"I suppose, but what would I do everyday while everyone else is outside for recess?" I asked.

"I don't know, but we could figure something out. What if we just worked on some fun stuff, like experiments or something?"

Knowing that Mr. Stensgard enjoyed teaching science as much as I enjoyed learning about it, I instantly became excited. "Do you think we could do experiments? Different science experiments?" I asked, obviously excited.

"You bet, we could try some experiments, work ahead in your math. We can meet and look through different topics that interest you, and try to develop experiments."

"Oh wow! This is going to be so cool!" I said.

"Yeah, I think it will be," Mr. Stensgard said with a big smile on his face.

For the rest of sixth grade I worked with Mr. Stensgard during recess on different projects. We would meet and determine what subject we were interested in looking into for the next few weeks, and then he would find materials for me to use to research our topic. Once I had researched a topic Mr. Stensgard would help me develop a few experiments to test my theories, and try to reinforce the ideas I had just completed researching. The topics of study ranged from density tests (using different objects to see how much water they displaced from a water bath) to conservation of momentum to gravity experiments.

Over the course of a few weeks, working only during recess, Mr. Stensgard also taught me basic algebra and gave me an introduction into trigonometry. Because of the time I spent working with Mr. Stensgard over recess for the second half of sixth grade, the majority of my math and science lessons over the next two years were a review for me.

Fontan Revisited

As sixth grade finished and the summer before Junior High started, I still did not know what was happening with my heart. I had been back to Dr. Stone's office several times and undergone several tests. I walked on a treadmill while Dr. Stone monitored my heart. I walked until I was pretty sure I was either going to pass out or vomit. I was shocked and disappointed when I realized that I had only spent a few minutes walking on the treadmill before I was unable to continue.

Dr. Stone ordered several other tests to further study what was happening with my heart. I wore a heart monitor that was fed into a recorder that I wore on my belt. The monitor looked like an oversized Walkman, which I wore everyday for several days. The tape was brought back to Dr. Stone so he could see what my heart had been doing during the course of an average day.

The final test at the end of the summer was the most invasive testing procedure. Dr. Stone ordered an angiogram to look at my heart and measure the pressures within each chamber of the heart. During the angiogram, the doctors sedated me heavily and then put a catheter tube into the vein in my groin. The catheter was fed up the vein and into my heart. Once the tip of the catheter reaches the heart, the doctor inflates a balloon on the end of the catheter to measure the pressures inside the heart.

In order to see the catheter and direct its movement, an X-ray dye is released from the catheter into the blood. As that blood was pumped from my heart throughout my body I could feel the heat of the dye spreading all over. Instantly I broke out into a sweat, and as my lungs were warmed by the dye, my body was tricked into thinking I was not getting enough oxygen. Dr. Stone told me to relax as I struggled and gasped for breath. Quickly the dye dissipated and the warm feeling left along with it.

When the test was completed and the catheter was removed, two large nurses applied direct pressure to my groin in an attempt to stop the bleeding from the major blood vessel. After several minutes of the crushing pressure from the nurses, their hands were replaced by a large sand bag laid across my thigh on top of the pressure bandage.

When I finally started to feel sleepy and groggy from the drugs given me earlier to sedate me for the tests, everything was complete and I was wheeled into the recovery room. Dr. Stone met with my parents and me after the angiogram to tell us the procedure had gone fine. The results would be studied in the next few days. After a few hours in the recovery room to ensure the bandage on my thigh was holding, I was discharged from the hospital.

My parents and I kept very busy the following week while we waited for the results of the angiogram. I spent every day with my dad volunteering at a fundraiser in Elk River. That summer the Elk River Police Department, along with local businesses, developed a plan to build a house in seven days with donated labor and materials. Once completed the house was sold, with all the proceeds going to the Drug Abuse

Resistance Education program that placed police officers in the schools to teach children to stay away from drugs.

Each day I went with my dad to the building site and helped out in any way I could. I brought the workers tools and refreshments. I spent hours following around the construction workers, picking up nails and scrap lumber. On the final day as the finishing touches were being done to the house, the final ribbon cutting ceremony was being put into place. I was stringing the ribbon across the front door when my dad asked me to come over to him. I walked over to my dad, who was standing outside our car talking on his car phone. As I approached, he said good-bye to the person on the other end of the phone and handed the receiver to me.

"Hello?" I said as I grabbed the phone.

"Hi, honey. How are you?" asked my mom, her voice trembling. As she spoke, my dad, who was standing behind, reached around me and began to hug me.

"Mom, what's wrong?" I asked immediately.

"Well, Dr. Stone called, Nick…" As my mom began I could feel the color draining from my face. I began to cry as she continued to speak. "…I know, honey. I know. Dr. Stone called and said we are going to have to schedule surgery." I cried harder as I heard the word surgery. She continued, "I know, we are going to have to be tough. We are going to have to get through this again."

"I know, Mom, I know," I whispered into the phone.

"We all kind of knew this was probably what he was going to say," she said.

"No, I know. But…but…it's just…it's still hard to hear it," I tried to explain.

"I know, honey, I know," she said, comforting me.

"Nick, do you want me to take you home quick?" my dad asked.

"Yeah," Mom said through the phone. "Nick, have Dad drive you home."

"No, the house is done," I said. "I want to stay for the opening ceremony."

"Are you sure?" asked my dad. "How about I bring you home? You don't need to stay for this. You have helped a lot already."

"I know, I want to stay for the end. Can I please stay?"

"Yes, of course you can," my dad said as he squeezed me with a big hug.

"Okay. Well, I am going to stay here, Mom. Thank you, I love you."

"Bye, Hon," she said.

"Bye, Mom."

Less than a half-hour after that conversation I went with my dad back over to the site of the new house for the opening ceremony. I was asked to cut the ribbon on the DARE house during the ceremony. I stood in front of everyone and pushed all the thoughts about surgery out of my mind. I smiled big for the cameras and cut the ribbon.

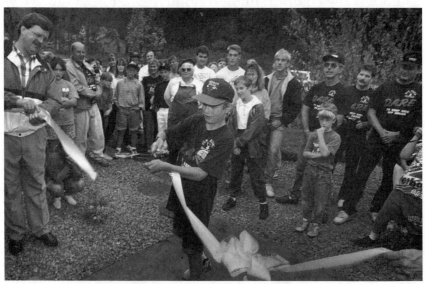

Nick cutting ribbon at DARE house

A few weeks later, in preparation for the first day of school at VandenBerge Junior High, my dad took me to the school to introduce me to a few people. My dad had set up a meeting with the principal of the school, Ron Gaarder, and the assistant principal, Jim Weinman, to discuss a few specifics about attending junior high. Mr. Gaarder told my dad and me that I probably should go in between classes using a wheelchair since the school was so spread out. A friend could push me around in the wheelchair from class to class, but he recommended that we leave class a few minutes early in order to avoid the congestion in the hallways.

Mr. Gaarder explained that I was scheduled to be in gym class with Mrs. Conley every morning during fall semester. He introduced us to her, and she was very nice. She listened to our concerns about gym class, and what I would and would not be able to participate in. Mrs. Conley recommended that while I was recovering from my heart surgery scheduled for November, that I work with her husband, Dave Conley, who worked in the In School Suspension (ISS) room. Mr. Conley taught ninth grade health and ran the ISS room at VandenBerge Junior High. A few years earlier he had coronary bypass surgery.

The first day of seventh grade I began school like every other seventh grader that morning, a little apprehensive about starting junior high school. My concerns probably differed considerably from the rest of the students, however. My best friend and next-door neighbor, Ryan Ebert, was there with me that morning. He went with me into the nurse's office to get the wheelchair I would be riding in. That morning Ryan had the task of not only finding his way to his classes on time, but finding my classes as well. Ryan wheeled me to every one of my classes, then he went to his next class for every period of the school day. He followed that routine everyday until I left school for my surgery.

When I arrived at Minneapolis Children's Hospital I was really surprised by what I saw as I walked into the lobby. A large group of people was sitting along the walls in the main entrance of the hospital as I walked in. I started recognizing the people in the lobby as my aunts and uncles, cousins, neighbors, and friends. It was shortly before 5:00 A.M. I was just arriving for my preoperative check-in time, and these people were already there. I had a few minutes to talk with most of them and thank everyone for their support. Shortly after I arrived at the hospital it was time for my family and I to meet with the doctors.

My parents, Tommy, David, and I all waited together in a small room for Dr. Stone. The nurses had already gotten me changed into a pair of hospital scrubs and had given me some medication to help relax. As I sat on the hospital bed visiting with my brothers, Dr. Stone came into the room. Instantly everybody stopped talking, and turned their attention towards him. I smiled and greeted Dr. Stone warmly. "Good morning, Dr. Stone. Are you ready to get this show on the road?" I joked.

"Good morning, Nick," Dr. Stone chuckled, and then turned his attention to the whole family. "Okay, lets go over briefly what Dr. Nicoloff is going to do in today's surgery. This is a redo of the Fontan procedure, and in the surgery we will be replacing the human aorta homograph with a synthetic gortex material tube. Now, this surgery may last longer due to the issues with scar tissue we have discussed before. The scar tissue formed in Nick's chest may complicate the surgery, requiring Dr. Nicoloff to work slowly to open Nick's chest. What Dr. Nicoloff is concerned about is the lungs actually being adhered to the chest wall. This would greatly complicate opening Nick's chest, and may make damage to his lungs more of a possibility. Now, those are our concerns. On the upside, replacing the homograph with the gortex conduit will greatly improve the flow into Nick's lungs. Hopefully Nick will be feeling good as new again soon."

Everyone shook their heads in agreement with Dr. Stone, hoping I would be feeling well again soon. My mom looked up at Dr. Stone and asked, "When will we know if the scar tissue is causing a problem with the surgery and his lungs?"

"We won't know if it really is a problem unless something happens and it causes some problems," he replied. "There are lots of things going on in any surgery, scar tissue is one factor. Don't get hung up on any one thing."

Dr. Stone stood up and turned his attention towards me. "Okay, I am going to go get ready for you," he said as he patted me on the head. "I will see you back there in a few minutes."

Shortly after Dr. Stone left the room a nurse entered to tell my parents that she would be bringing me back to the operating room in a few minutes. I looked around the room, able to make out my parents and brothers, although I was having trouble focusing on any one thing. The relaxation medication was causing me to smile and ramble on in near incoherent conversations. My brother Tommy was the first one to sit next to me on my bed, followed shortly by David. They sat next to me and leaned in, draping their arms around me, and began talking.

"Nick, stay strong. We are all here for you. You just have to stay strong and fight," Tommy began.

"Nick, we love you. You can do this. You're the strongest person I know, and I know you can do this. We just love you so much," Dave whispered.

"I know, I know. I love you, too. I love you guys, too." I started to speak, but was unable to continue talking through the tears.

Tommy squeezed tightly and said, "We love you so much, and we need you to make it through this. You have to keep fighting."

"I will, Tommy. I will be okay," I said in a convincing voice.

My parents joined the huddle, putting their arms around Tommy and David. They rubbed Tommy and David's backs as they were draped around me. Tommy and David continued crying as my parents began to speak.

"Nick, look at how much your big brothers love you. They are so close to you. We all love you, honey. We all love you so much," Mom said softly.

"Bud, just keep fighting. Never ever give up, Nick, just keep fighting," my dad begged.

As my family continued to hug me, the nurse came into the room and announced it was time for me to be taken into the operating room. Everyone gave me their final words of encouragement and last hugs. Tommy held on to me, seemingly unwilling to release his grip. My dad grabbed Tommy by his shoulders and pulled him off the bed.

"Son, son, its time. You have to let him go," Dad said.

"No. No. Not yet, not yet," Tommy wailed loudly.

I looked back at my family as I was being wheeled out of the room. I smiled and said, "Hey, don't worry about me. Everything is going to be fine, everything will work out fine. I will see you soon."

My parents took Tommy and David directly to the hospital chapel to pray for strength. They stayed in the chapel a long time, knelt in prayer and silently reflected on the continued challenge before their family. After the prayers were said, and some more tears were shed, the family went back to the surgical waiting room. In the waiting room, extended family, neighbors, friends, and coworkers of my parents still continued to hold vigil. Some told stories, a few told jokes, but most kept occupied reading, simply waiting on news.

Shortly into their wait, my family and friends were shocked to see Dr. Stone enter the room. He approached my parents and asked to speak to them privately. Instantly panicked by Dr. Stone's reserved body language, my mom began to cry. My dad tried to comfort her as they walked into an adjoining consultation room with Dr. Stone. Once in the private room, Dr. Stone explained that their son was still alive, but something had gone terribly wrong. While Dr. Nicoloff made the incision with the saw through the breastbone, the scar tissue in Nick's chest had complicated things. Because of the adhesion of the scar tissue, the lungs and the heart were actually attached to the chest wall. While Dr. Nicoloff cut through Nick's chest with the saw, the saw cut through Nick's heart.

Dr. Stone explained the team was able to finish opening Nick's chest and hook him up to the bypass machine in less than thirty seconds. Massive amounts of blood products had been infused to replace the blood volume lost in this complication. The rest of the surgery could still be completed, but the complication would likely cause the surgery to take even longer. Dr. Stone then excused himself from the room in order to get back to the operating room.

My parents, still in shock by the news Dr. Stone had delivered, went into the main waiting room and calmed the fears of their friends and family. They explained there had been a complication and that Nick's heart was cut while his chest was being opened. However, the damage had been repaired, and the blood that was lost had already been replaced.

Waking up from surgery is always a little bewildering. The pain medications and remnants from the anesthesia don't allow you to awake all at once. Instead, you drift in and out of consciousness, acutely aware of some things, and undeniably oblivious to others. My parents were constantly near me in the Intensive Care Unit at Minneapolis Children's Hospital. Both Tommy and David were constantly close as well, everyone rotating to ensure people got breaks, and I was never alone. For hours they would sit in a chair along my bedside, hunched forward and holding my hand or rubbing my arm. For hours they kept up this routine, so that once every few hours when I did wake for a short period of time, I was never alone.

I was not afraid as I woke up this time like I was several years earlier. I was almost a teenager, like an adult, I thought.

When I woke up and heard the ventilator breathing for me, I was comforted. I was frustrated about not being able to talk, and again I would have traded anything for a drink of juice. However, I was more patient this time around. I wrote conversations on a note pad with different visitors and constantly gave a thumbs-up to those in the room.

Within twelve hours after surgery, the ventilator tube was removed from my throat, and I was again breathing on my own. I was delighted to moisten my throat with ice chips and little sips of fruit punch. It was a relief to everyone in the following days after surgery when it was apparent that my other vocal chord suffered no damage in this surgery. One concern going into another heart surgery so similar to the previous surgery was nerve damage to the remaining functional vocal chord, rendering me mute. That was thankfully not the case; I was able to talk nonstop to my nurses and all of my visitors.

My Grandma Helga stayed with me all night so Mom and Dad could try and sleep in the parents' room. Grandma loved doing the "night shift" and never missed one night during my stays in intensive care.

A few days after surgery I was sitting in a chair next to my hospital bed, enjoying my first meal after surgery (it was supposed to be scrambled eggs), when a doctor from Dr. Nicoloff's surgical group came in my room. He told me he was there to remove the two drainage tubes from my chest tubes.

"No! You are not coming near me until I have meds!" I said very sternly as I pushed my nurse's button.

"Nick, let's just pull these tubes out quick and we will be done with it," the surgeon replied.

Remembering all too clearly my experience with chest tubes six years earlier, I stood my ground. "You are not pulling out my tubes until I have pain medication and the medication has had time to take effect."

"What do you need, Nick?" the nurse asked as she entered the room, unaware of the confrontation that was brewing.

"I need to remove Nick's chest tube. Now!" The surgeon told the nurse.

"Nothing is being pulled until I have some pain medication," I repeated.

"Okay…let me get something for you, Nick," the nurse said as she left the room.

She retrieved some pain medication and quickly administered the drugs. She sat by my side for a while, and then began preparing the materials needed to remove the chest tubes. After sufficiently stalling the doctor so the medication would have time to begin working, she smiled and looked at the surgeon and said, "Looks like we are all ready now." My nurses were always my advocates.

The surgeon, resigned to having already lost this struggle, simply said, "Thank you." He removed the tape from around the tubes and instructed me briefly on how to breathe as he removed the tubes. On the count of three I could feel him pulling at the tubes. My body wretched and braced for the onslaught of pain. However, the pain did not come as I felt the tubes worm their way out of my body. Stunned, I looked around in shock, and then in disbelief I asked the surgeon, "Are they already out?"

The surgeon cracked a smile, tilted his head and said, "See, I told you it wouldn't hurt." He then patted me on the back and said, "Nick, you did great." As he left I overheard him thank the nurse for her patience with him, and for working so quickly.

This instance was the first time in my life I acted as an advocate on my own behalf. As a twelve-year-old boy, I stood up to a distinguished surgeon. I demanded that my needs be met by him, and insisted that I be provided the best possible care. My nurse that morning was a tremendous help to slow down the doctor for just a few minutes to allow the pain medication to take effect.

Just seven days after my surgery I was discharged from Minneapolis Children's Hospital. As I settled into my routine at home recovering from the surgery, my junior high principal, Mr. Gaarder, arranged for a homeschool teacher to visit my home and teach me a few hours each day. With the help and support of my parents and teachers, I was able to make up nearly a month and a half of missed schoolwork from seventh grade. A few weeks before Christmas break, I returned to school at VandenBerge Junior High with the rest of my friends. My best friend, Ryan Ebert, again pushed my wheelchair to all of my classes for the next month.

A few weeks after starting back to class, for the first time I began getting into my own as a junior high student. I was able to move about on my own, meet new people, and for the first time in a year and a half I had the energy to do everything I wanted to do. Prior to the surgery I was choosing between being active and feeling well. After returning to school, I joined some of the student groups I didn't have the energy to participate in earlier. For the rest of seventh grade I was able to attend school and participate like any other normal junor high student.

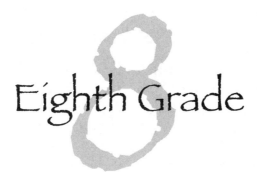

Eighth Grade

"Nick, we have been working on this speech for quite a while. Do you want to take a break yet?" Mom asked.

Just then the front door opened and my dad came in the house. "Hello, I'm home," he announced. "Have you two been working on that speech all afternoon?".

"Well, Dad, you know Mom always puts things off until the last minute," I teased.

"Me! Oh, yeah. You had an entire year to work on this speech. It's not my fault you didn't start working on it until the week before you graduate," she teased back.

"I am having a hard time believing you are actually graduating this weekend," my dad said through his smile. "Nick, we are just so proud of you."

"Well, I am proud of us," I said. "I wouldn't have made it through junior high without everyone's support. That's what I can't believe—I can't believe how many people put things in their lives on hold to help us while I was waiting for my surgery."

The start of eighth grade was a rude awakening for me. Over the summer I had not been nearly as active as during the final months of my seventh grade year. So, I was really surprised when I started back to school and noticed I was not physically able to do the things I had been doing before.

The realization that there was something wrong didn't occur to me for several months. The first few weeks of classes I was convinced my busy schedule was just keeping me worn out. Then, I seemed to catch a cold bug, and for the next month I attributed my sluggishness and queasiness to a flu bug I just couldn't shake. Finally, a few months into the fall semester, I became concerned that something else was going on. I wrestled with the idea that something was wrong with my heart for quite a while before I approached my parents.

One evening I walked into the living room where my parents were watching TV and sat on the couch. During a commercial break I turned, looked at my parents, and brought their world crashing in on them.

"Mom, Dad," I began stoically, "something is wrong again; I don't feel well," I said very authoritatively. "I don't know what it is, but I am pretty sure it's my heart…" My voice cracked as I trailed off.

"What do you mean?" my dad asked immediately.

"What do you mean, you don't feel well?" my mom echoed.

"I feel sick. Whenever I do anything I feel sick," I replied softly.

"How long have you been feeling sick?" my dad asked urgently.

"Well, a couple of months ago I noticed…"

"A couple of months ago!" my dad interrupted. "Nick, you need to tell us these things. You just can't keep us in the dark," he continued.

"I am telling you!" I snapped back. Feeling very defensive I said, "A couple of months ago, when school started, I felt worn down. Then I got that cold and I wasn't feeling very well. Time has passed, and I just never got better. I still can't do what I could last spring."

"What things are you talking about?" Mom asked.

"Its not that I physically can't do things, but when I do exert myself I feel sick. If I stand too long, or when I walk from class to class, I feel sick. I spend the first five to ten minutes in each class feeling exhausted and sick to my stomach," I explained.

"Nick, why didn't you tell us earlier?" Dad asked again.

"Dad," I began, turning my head and looking right at him, "because I just didn't know until now. As soon as I was sure, I came to you guys."

"Well, tomorrow we will get a hold of Dr. Stone and see how soon we can get you in," he said.

The following day I tried to concentrate on classes, but was not very successful. I walked slowly to my classes, drifting almost aimlessly down the hallways of the school. After I arrived at class, I sat at my desk and became lost in my thoughts. While my teachers discussed the previous night's reading assignment and today's lesson, I thought about being sick again. I couldn't believe that I had my fourth surgery less than a year earlier, and I already felt sick again. I thought about how much work it was to stay caught up on my schoolwork. But mostly, I couldn't stop thinking about what this was going to do to my family. Seeing my parents and my brothers struggle through my last surgery was very difficult on me. The thought of our lives being turned upside down for another surgery once again was devastating. My teacher interrupted my daydreaming. "Nick, Nick!" she repeated.

I looked up and noticed that she, along with nearly all of the students in my class, were staring at me. "What? What's up?" I stammered, trying to figure out why everyone was looking at me.

"Nick, you have a pass from the office," the teacher said, motioning towards the door.

"Oh, uh, yeah, okay," I said as I noticed the office runner standing in the doorway. Slowly I began to piece things together. I gathered my things and followed the student down to the office. My dad was in the main office waiting for me there. He signed me out of class, and we went outside to the parking lot. My dad's truck was parked along the curb, and my mom was waiting in the passenger seat. Dad explained that Dr. Stone told them to bring me into his office; he would see me today.

We didn't wait long before Dr. Stone called us back into one of the exam rooms. As he took my blood pressure he began asking me questions.

"Nick, when you say you aren't feeling well, what specifically do you mean by that?"

"Well, Dr. Stone, just going through my average day at school makes me feel worn down. I get tired out easily, and feel like I don't have enough energy to do the things I want to do."

"Okay, I see," he replied. He leaned in close to me as he placed his stethoscope on my chest.

"If I stand too long, walk too much, or do too much, I feel sick in my stomach. Then I feel like I can't get enough oxygen. Then I feel terrible for the rest of the afternoon, or until I lay down," I explained.

Dr. Stone was hunched forward next to me. He moved his stethoscope across my chest. He was silent, not even breathing as he listened. "Breathe in," he whispered. I drew in a deep breath. He stayed motionless for a few seconds, and then said, "Now breathe out." I exhaled as I was told to do. I looked over Dr. Stone's shoulder and noticed my parents watching closely. I could tell just by looking at them how nervous they were.

Dr. Stone sighed heavily as he sat upright and slid his chair back from the exam table. He swiveled his chair slightly to the right, looked at my parents, and said, "Well, I don't know what would be going on with Nick's heart, but I definitely want to look into it."

"Does anything look different from our last appointment?" my mom asked.

"Not that I can tell, but I am going to want to do a lot more tests before we can rule anything in or out," he explained.

Dr. Stone scheduled a few follow-up tests for me to undergo during the following days. He scheduled a cardiac stress test and an angiogram to measure the pressures in my heart, which he would view with the radioactive dye. He also gave me a heart monitor to wear home.

I returned to school the following day wearing the portable heart monitor. Knowing Dr. Stone was looking into what was wrong, I was able to once again focus on my classes. I didn't really confide in any of my friends about my new health concerns. I didn't want to unnecessarily alarm them, so I acted normal. I hid the wires from the heart monitor as best I could and made up excuses for not being as energetic as normal. As hard as I tried to keep things to myself, it wasn't long before people started asking me questions. I was able to deflect these for the most part; I just told people that I was really worn down and I didn't feel well.

I continued going to school with the heart monitor under my clothes for several weeks. My parents and I went down to Minneapolis Children's Hospital for the stress test. This stress test was similar to the others I had done. I climbed onto the treadmill and began walking steadily, focusing on breathing and keeping a steady pace. Like the stress tests I had done in the past, it was not long before I was feeling tired and sick. I breathed heavily, desperately trying to get oxygen into my body. My legs went numb, and I began to feel nauseous as I struggled to keep my legs moving forward. Before long I signaled to the doctors that I needed to stop, and as the whirring of the treadmill slowed I stepped off of the machine and struggled to climb up onto the exam table.

I laid flat on my back, staring at the ceiling above the table as the nurses and doctors scurried around me. They began taking blood pressure measurements and observed my heart with the ultrasound equipment. As they worked above me, I struggled to catch my breath and relieve the nauseating feeling that had enveloped my entire body. They continued to take readings and measurements for nearly a half hour after I had stopped walking on the treadmill. As they wrapped up their work Dr. Stone came to the head of the bed, where my parents were sitting next to me.

Dr. Stone grabbed my arm and looked over at my parents and said, "Well, it's pretty clear that Nick is having a problem with exercise tolerance. The next step is to get some pressure measurements from inside the heart."

"So, go ahead and schedule a heart cath?" my mom asked.

"Yes, I think an angiogram is the next step to find out what's going on inside Nick's heart. We will schedule the test through my office for sometime next week."

My parents and I all nodded our heads in agreement. Then I turned my head, looked at my parents, and said, "Well, at least it seems like we are making progress. The sooner they know what's wrong, the sooner they can fix it."

"Well, Nick," Dr. Stone said as he patted my leg, "we are going to work as hard as we can to figure out what is going wrong."

Dr. Stone instructed my parents to call the clinic and schedule the angiogram. He then excused himself from the room. As he gathered his files he looked at me and said, "Nick, I know this has been going on for a while now, and it looks like it will be a bit longer before we have any definite answers. As tough as it might be, you need to keep busy and stay active—don't worry yet. We don't even know what to be worried about yet."

"Okay, thank you, Dr. Stone," I replied quietly.

The following week I did my best to keep my mind on other things. At school I focused on the student groups I was involved with, along with a few end-of-the-semester projects I was trying to complete. As the days passed and the angiogram grew nearer, I found it more and more difficult to concentrate on my schoolwork. Mr. Gaarder, my junior high principal, passed me in the hallway one afternoon. He stopped and turned around to face me.

"Nick!" he said loudly. I turned around to face him abruptly. "Nick, come here," he said matter-of-factly. I quickly walked back towards the principal, trying to figure out what I had done to get into trouble.

"Nick, is everything all right?" he asked quietly.

"Uh, yeah, Mr. Gaarder. Everything is great," I replied, as enthusiastically as possible.

"Nick, come into my office. I would like to talk with you," he said with unmistakable empathy in his voice.

He walked briskly towards his office, and I followed closely behind him. As I tailed Mr. Gaarder, my mind raced, trying to figure out what he wanted to speak to me about. I tried desperately to figure out why he wanted me to go into his office for a talk with the principal. He turned around as we entered his office and said, "Shut the door behind you."

I looked at him, confused by his request. In disbelief I turned and shut the door of his office. He walked behind his desk and sat in his oversized chair.

"Nick, why don't you sit for a bit so we can talk," he ordered, more than he asked.

I sat down in the small chair on the opposite side of his desk, looked across the desk at him and asked, "So what's up?" I worked hard to keep my voice as upbeat as possible.

"Nick, is everything going all right?" he asked once again.

"Yeah, Mr. Gaarder. School is going great," I replied honestly.

"I know. I know things at school are going well for you. What about other things? How are you feeling?"

"Oh, fine," I said immediately. Mr. Gaarder instantly gave me a disapproving look, and I continued, "Well, what I mean is, I am doing fine, but I have been feeling tired lately. I have been sick, and I am pretty sure it's a flu bug or something…"

"Nick," Mr. Gaarder began, cutting me off mid sentence, "your father called me this morning. I know you aren't feeling well. I know you have been seeing your cardiologist."

"Oh," I said, instantly feeling guilty about lying to Mr. Gaarder.

"Nick. How are you feeling?" he asked for the third time.

"Mr. Gaarder, I don't feel good at all. I know something is wrong with my heart again. The doctors are doing lots of tests to try to figure it out. My parents are hoping I don't have to have another surgery, but I know I will," I blurted out quickly. As I spoke I could feel the lump form in my throat and tears welling in my eyes.

"Nick, you can't pretend like everything is fine when you are going through this. You need to be honest with people," Mr. Gaarder said as he moved his chair from behind his desk.

"I know and I will be," I began, "but I need to know what's going on before I talk to people. As soon as people know that I am sick again, that's all they will talk about. I work really hard not to think about this every minute of every day. But then my dad has people talking to me about it, and asking me how I feel." As I spoke my voice trailed off, and I began to cry. "Mr. Gaarder," I said after I cleared my throat, "when I am ready to talk about it I will, but I want to know what I am dealing with first."

"Nick, if there is anything, anything I can do, please, just let me know what you need," he said softly.

"Thank you. Thank you for talking to me today. I know that you and Mr. Conley are always there if I need something, and that is a big help," I said as I stood up.

"We are, Nick. So, if you need something, just be sure to let us know," he replied.

On the morning of the heart cath, my parents and I arrived at Minneapolis Children's Hospital at 7:00 A.M. We checked in and registered, and were taken back into the pre-op area. The nurse prepping me for the heart cath gave me a little Versed in my IV to help sedate me for the procedure. My parents and I were visiting and talking about school, trying to make small talk about anything other than today's test. The nurse opened the curtain surrounding my bed and told us that I had a phone call at the nurses' station. Surprised, I sat up to walk to the nurses' station, but because I had been given a sedative already the nurse would not allow me out of bed. Instead, she wheeled my bed close to the nurses' desk and handed me the telephone receiver. My parents were curious as to who would be calling me in the pre-op area this early in the morning.

"Hello?" I said, bringing the phone next to my ear.

"Nick?" said a familiar voice on the other end of the line.

"Yes?" I replied, still unsure of the caller's identity.

"Nick, this is Ron Gaarder and Dave Conley calling from VandenBerge," Mr. Gaarder said.

"Oh, Mr. Gaarder. Hello, sir. How are you this morning?" I said, speaking very slowly.

"Uh, we are fine, Nick. We were actually calling to see how you were doing this morning."

"Oh, I feel great!" I said loudly into the phone.

"Okay. Well, Nick, we just wanted to get a hold of you this morning to wish you luck, and let you know that all of us here are thinking about you and praying for you."

"Mr. Gaarder, Mr. Conley, thank you, I really appreciate everything you have done for me," I said.

As I hung up the phone I noticed my mom was crying and speaking to my father. She was shaking her head as she spoke, with a large smile across her face.

"Mom? What's wrong? Why are you crying?" I asked.

"No, honey. I am just...I just can't believe your principal and your teacher called the hospital and tracked you down at the nurses' station. And that they called to wish you luck, and told you that they were praying for you. You have touched so many lives in so many different ways. It's just amazing," she said.

Shortly after the phone call the nurse came over to my bed and told us that they were ready for me in the cath lab. I hugged my parents and told them I would see them in a little while. I waved to my parents, and as my bed began rolling through a maze of hallways to the cath lab, I closed my eyes and drifted to sleep.

Several times during the heart cath I groggily woke up. I could feel Dr. Stone manipulating the catheter through the blood vessel in my groin and up into my chest. As the catheter released the radioactive dye, I felt a warm wave come over my entire body. My chest felt like it was on fire as the dye worked its way through my heart and lungs.

As Dr. Stone wrapped up my heart cath he walked up to the head of my bed. He leaned forward next to my face and said, "Nick, you did great, just like you do every time. The nurses are going to get you settled into the recovery area, and I will be in there to see you in a little bit."

As the catheter was removed from the blood vessel in my groin, two nurses began applying direct pressure to quell the bleeding, and soon these two full-grown adults were kneeling on top of the sand bag placed on my lap to provide more pressure to stop the bleeding. In disbelief of the amount of pain coming from the small incision site the nurses were now kneeling on, I tried with little success to fall back asleep. Close to fifteen minutes later when the bleeding had finally subsided, the nurses transported me back to the recovery area.

I was laying in the recovery room drifting in and out of sleep when Dr. Stone came through the door. As he approached my bed I immediately knew there was something different about him. His face looked slightly tense, and he appeared very tired. I sat up slightly in bed and asked, "Well, Dr. Stone, what's the plan? Do we know what's going on in there yet?"

"Nick, there is nothing we can do," Dr. Stone said, looking down at me. "The right side of your heart is severely enlarged and is unable to pump blood to your lungs. The blood is entering that right atrium and swirling around, and the atrium is so large it is unable to forcefully pump the blood out."

"Oh, well. How do we fix that?" I asked. As I spoke I could feel a pit in my stomach growing.

"Nick, we can't fix it. We can't repair your heart this time. I am going to refer you across the street to Abbott Northwestern Hospital's heart transplant program. Nick, you need a heart transplant." When he finished speaking he looked very upset; he abruptly turned around and walked out of the recovery unit.

Absolutely stunned, there was nothing I could do but cry. I lay in the hospital bed and cried. My tears grew to sobs, and my sobbing progressed to wailing. My nurse, unaware of the news I had received from Dr. Stone, asked if I was in pain, and checked the catheter site to ensure it had not reopened. After a while I ran out of energy to cry, and simply fell asleep.

When I woke from my nap my parents were sitting next to my bed. My mom was rubbing my arm, and my dad was rubbing my head. My mom leaned forward and said, "Nick, you did so good, and you were so brave."

Unable to bring myself to tell them the news Dr. Stone had given me, I simply said nothing. I remained almost completely silent until after I had been checked out of the hospital later that day. I was in the back seat of my parent's truck, and my mom began talking about our appointment the next day at Dr. Stone's office.

"Nick, whatever Dr. Stone says tomorrow, just remember we have made it this far together as a family, and we will keep going," she said, her voice cracking slightly as she spoke.

My dad stared straight ahead, saying almost as little as I had after Dr. Stone talked to me earlier that day.

My mom continued, "No matter what Dr. Stone says tomorrow, we just have to stick together and keep fighting as a family. Together, it doesn't matter what it is, we can get through it. If another surgery is needed we will make it through, if something else needs to be done, we can do that, too."

As I heard my mom talk about another surgery, or something else, I slumped back into the back seat, and began quietly crying. My mom looked back at me and asked, "Nick, what's wrong? Why are you crying?"

"Dr. Stone talked to me after the heart cath, before you guys were there." I began crying harder as I spoke. "…And Dr. Stone told me he couldn't do anything. Mom, he said I need a heart transplant."

My mom turned completely around in the front seat of the car and reached back towards me. "Nick," she began, "Dr. Stone talked to dad and me, too. We know what he found out. Nick, we are going to get through this."

"Why didn't you guys talk to me when you came back to see me? Why didn't you tell me you knew?" I asked.

"We didn't think you knew yet. You seemed upset, and we didn't want to tell you. We were going to wait for the meeting at Dr. Stone's office tomorrow morning," she said. "Why didn't you tell us that you had talked to Dr. Stone?"

"When you guys came back to recovery you seemed so happy that everything went well. I couldn't bring myself to tell you that Dr. Stone said there was nothing he could do," I explained.

"Nick, Tom, these next few months are going to be hard on us all. We need to be there for each other like we always have been in the past. We can't keep things from each other as a way to protect ourselves. I think we need to be honest, open and up front. Look how upset we all have been today. All of us upset by the news Dr. Stone gave us, and we all kept that inside, and refused to talk about it, because it might hurt someone else. So, what did we do? We all hurt separately from the same news, but we couldn't rely on each other," my mom explained.

"Nick, your mom is right. Sitting here thinking about this, acting like everything is okay, doesn't help anyone. I am sorry we didn't talk to you right away," Dad said.

"Guys, I am sorry, too. I lay in bed silently, moping. That didn't make me feel any better. I should have just talked to you guys. I am sorry," I said.

The next morning my parents and I met with Dr. Stone at his office in Minneapolis. Dr. Stone explained to my parents and me once again what was wrong with my heart. During the Fontan surgery I had when I was seven years old, my heart was redesigned so the right atrium pumped the blood to my lungs. Forcing the right atrium to do much more work then it was originally designed to do caused the atrium to enlarge and become sluggish. The enlarged right atrium allowed blood to pool, and did not create enough pressure to effectively pump blood to my lungs.

Dr. Stone explained this was not a problem that could be fixed by adjusting the mechanics of my heart, because the heart muscle itself was too weak. The atrium had enlarged so much that it would be impossible to effectively pump blood. That was why there was no surgical alternative, and the enlarged heart had to be replaced. Dr. Stone made an appointment for me at Abbott Northwestern Hospital's heart transplant program with Dr. Marc Pritzker.

"You Need A Heart Transplant"

The process a patient has to go through to be placed on the heart transplant waiting list was more involved then my parents and I could have possibly imagined. All of my medical files were first forwarded to the transplant group to be evaluated. Once that evaluation was complete, several days of appointments were scheduled with different members of the transplant group.

"All right, Nick, you and your parents can have a seat in here, and wait," said Mary O'Kane, the transplant coordinator. "The people wishing to speak to you will be in and out throughout the day." My parents and I sat in the small room and waited. We passed the time by joking with each other and trying to keep entertained. It wasn't long before I was rummaging through the drawers in the small exam room.

"Mom," I said, turning around to face her. "What do you think the psychologist would say if he walked in now?" I had cotton balls stuffed up my nose and a tongue depressor hanging out of my mouth.

"Nicholas! Stop that! We can't let them know we are crazy," my mom laughed as she scolded me. Still laughing she continued, "We have to act sane, so they put you on the list. One day we have to fool them."

Just then someone knocked on the office door. My mom exaggerated a "Shhh…" sound to me and we both giggled as the man entered the room. He smiled warmly to all of us and sat down in the one empty chair. He introduced himself as a chaplain from the hospital. He began to explain some of the emotional and spiritual stresses people endure while waiting for a heart transplant. He talked about how difficult it can be on a family to receive so much joy in the form of a newly transplanted organ when there is such a deep loss from the family who donated the heart. He asked us quite a bit about our thoughts of a higher power and the existence of some type of divine control. After speaking with my parents and me, the chaplain talked about some of our coping strategies. In talking with us for less than forty-five minutes, he was able to tell how we rely on humor to cope with difficult situations and how we approached the future with a one-day-at-a-time mentality.

When our meeting with the chaplain had finished and he left the room, I immediately turned to my mom and said in an overly sneaky voice, "Okay, one down. Keep up the act, and we will be able to fool them all." We laughed and continued along with our running joke until the knock on the door brought us back to reality.

The next man to enter the room and interview us was an infectious disease specialist. This specialist had a laundry list of questions for me. Nearly all of them I was easily able to answer, although it was still very embarrassing as a fourteen-year-old to have an adult ask you about your sexual experiences (or lack of them in my case) in front of my parents. He also inquired about IV drug habits and exposure to exotic diseases. There were even several questions about my exposure to animals, such as monkeys and bats. After he was finished with his questions and had left it did not take long for my mom to start teasing me.

"So, Nick," she began, "how long has been it since you had sexual intercourse with an IV drug-using primate?"

I laughed so hard a sizeable amount of the apple juice I was drinking came out of my nose. Both of my parents erupted in laughter as I scrambled to find some paper towels to clean up my mess.

"You know what would be really funny?" my mom asked us.

"What?" my father and I replied in unison.

"What if the real tests weren't the people coming in and interviewing us? What if the room has a hidden camera, and they just studied how you act after each person leaves," she said.

"Well, if that were the case, then I think we are outta luck. They would watch this and be saying to each other, 'Oh, my God! This family is totally nuts!'" I laughed.

"Yeah, if that were the case, they would have had security throw us out by now," my dad joined in.

The knock at the door once again brought us away from our distraction. The woman who entered introduced herself as a social worker. She explained she was mainly interested in identifying the support structure in place to help me through the process of waiting for a transplant and managing my new heart post-transplant. She discussed some of the life-altering effects of organ transplant, including some new lifestyle limitations. It wasn't long before both of my parents were telling the social worker my entire life story, and how we had arrived to this point. My dad explained how my mom was my biggest support while I was sick. My mom talked about how my dad worked and took care of my older brothers, and then would come down to the hospital to be with us. I focused on the relationship I had with both of my parents, and on the open, honest communication.

When my parents were finished telling the social worker the complete history of my life and my family, I was shocked when I looked at her. She was holding a box of Kleenex in her lap, wiping the tears from her face. For some reason it didn't surprise me that the woman meeting with us to make sure we could handle the emotional stress of this situation was sobbing.

A few more specialists from various psychosocial disciplines sat down with the three of us that afternoon. My parents explained to each one of them how close our family was and how much we all rely on each other. My mother told stories about me struggling through school and always being sick. They both talked about our family pulling together, surviving off the strength of each other.

When the final interview of the day finished, relieved that the emotional day was finally past, we immediately continued our earlier joke about a hidden camera watching us. My mom and dad laughed as I acted out a mock reaction of the doctors watching us. I walked out of the doctor's office after one of the most stressful days of my life laughing so hard my stomach hurt.

Our next appointment with the transplant group was with the head transplant doctor, Dr. Marc Pritzker. Dr. Pritzker is truly a commanding presence in a room. He carries himself with an air of confidence I would imagine a general having while leading his troops to certain victory. Dr. Pritzker talked constantly and loudly. It didn't take long for a patient to realize during an appointment with him that you weren't going to say much. Dr. Pritzker often asked questions aloud, seemingly so he could answer them.

Dr. Pritzker's interpersonal skills aside, it became quickly apparent that the man was brilliant. His confidence and broad depth of knowledge instilled confidence in his patients, even if they didn't particularly care for him.

After the meetings with the specialists and with Dr. Pritzker, we were informed I was eligible and a good candidate for a heart transplant. The transplant coordinator, Mary

O'Kane, informed my parents that I would be placed on the heart transplant waiting list through Abbott Northwestern Hospitals transplant program. To insure I was always reachable by the transplant program I was given a pager to carry around with me.

I returned to school that winter after I was placed on the transplant wait list. When I started back to school that winter, my friend Ryan once again volunteered to push my wheelchair. Word spread quickly throughout the school I was once again sick. Rumors were more common than the truth. I spent most of my time assuring people that I didn't already have a heart transplant.

As the school year continued and students at VandenBerg Junior High once again became used to seeing me in a wheelchair, things began to return back to normal. However, things were anything but normal for me. I slowly began to realize the turn my life had taken when I wasn't paying attention. Gradually my life shifted beneath me, and at first I didn't even realize it. My friends were making plans for the Spring Formal Dance, just a month and a half away. I tried to think that far ahead in my life. I tried desperately to plan some fun things for a few months away. Every time I tried, all I could think about was whether or not I would still be waiting for a new heart.

Mr. Gaarder allowed me to rearrange my schedule for the remainder of the eighth grade year, since a gym class didn't really make much sense for me. Instead of gym class, Mr. Gaarder had me work with Mr. Conley an hour a day in the In School Suspension room. For an hour a day, Mr. Conley and I would joke about different things, and visit. I would help him with paperwork and try to help some of the students with their class work. Mr. Conley would go out of his way to keep the mood lighthearted and fun. Mr. Gaarder and Mr. Conley provided me an hour every day that spring to lift my spirits.

As my eighth grade year at VandenBerg Junior High came to an end, I was finding it more and more difficult to focus on school and homework. With the final days of class approaching, I began dreading summer vacation. I understood that once summer arrived I would not be able to see many of my friends until the following fall. I was having difficulty leaving home, even if I was going to be sitting in a wheelchair. Every day I grew more and more tired, and I was able to do less and less. I realized simple things like walking to a friend's house or going out to a movie were no longer going to be possible.

During the ice cream social at school that marked the last day of class, I would not let myself think about what nearly every one of my friends was thinking as they signed my yearbook. As they wrote notes in the back of my yearbook and gave me prolonged hugs and wiped a few tears from their eyes as they walked away from our goodbye, it was obvious many of them believed they would never see me again.

As I spoke with my friends that afternoon, I reassured them that I would see them over the summer and the following fall. In the final hours of class that afternoon, I struggled with how to say goodbye to my friends while maintaining my composure. The final bell signaled the end of the school year, and the students in my class cheered as they dashed out of the classroom. I sat in the nearly empty classroom, reluctant to leave. I thanked my teacher for her help and understanding during the year, before Ryan arrived to push my wheelchair out of the classroom. I left school reluctantly that afternoon, fearful of what the summer would bring.

The next few weeks really dragged on for me. I tried to talk with my friends on the phone as much as possible, but most of them had very busy, fun-filled summers going on. Some had summer jobs, others had family commitments, and a few of my friends simply found something fun to do everyday. My days revolved around what television programs were on TV, and with my mom home during the day, I watched a lot of soap operas and Oprah.

The Elk River Lion's Club, a local charity, approached my dad and asked what they could do to help me out. A member of the club, Les Anderson, had been following my story very closely for several years and wanted to do something to help ease the wait for a heart transplant. My dad explained how frustrated I had become because I was no longer healthy enough to walk to a friend's house, or even just leave the house and get around my neighborhood.

Les talked to some of the other Lion's Club members, and within a few weeks they had developed a plan to donate a golf cart to me that could be used to get me around my neighborhood for as long as I needed it. Les drove to our home and delivered the golf cart personally.

From that moment on my summer had changed. I was no longer unable to venture out of the house. The cart allowed me the freedom to visit my friends in the neighborhood and to be able to get to the park near our home. It gave me a renewed sense of mobility, freedom, and independence.

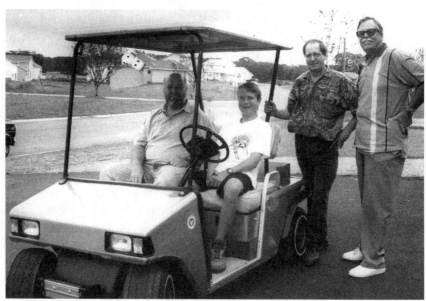

Nick in golf cart donated by the Lion's Club. Lion's Club members from left to right: Jim Mulroy, Ken Sinkler and Les Anderson

Ninth Grade—Just When There's Normalcy

Later that summer I met Karin at a friend's birthday party. Karin was a year older than me; she was about to begin school at Elk River High School. Throughout August, a month before school started, Karin and I spoke on the phone nearly every day. We would spend hours talking back and forth even when we had nothing to say. We would meet some evenings at the movie theater in town and watch a movie together. It is safe to say Karin was my first real girlfriend. I talked with her pretty openly about having a heart condition and being sick. She was always very understanding and very compassionate.

I knew she didn't quite understand the seriousness of my heart problem and what undergoing a heart transplant would involve, but that was one of the things I appreciated about being with her. When Karin and I spent time together, I was able to take my mind off everything else. I didn't worry about finding a match, I didn't focus on waiting, and I was content with just spending time with her.

While summer wound down, I started looking forward to my final year at VandenBerg Junior High. I couldn't wait to start back at school with all of my friends and be surrounded by people again. By the end of summer I truly missed being with people my age, and I was looking forward to keeping myself busy with class. During the summer, since I didn't have schoolwork and other teenagers to occupy a lot of my time, I found myself thinking about my heart transplant nearly everyday. I was looking forward to getting back into the rhythm of school, keeping busy with class, and being able to push my wait for a new heart into the back of my mind.

On the first day of my ninth grade year I arrived to school early with Ryan, and he pushed me through the hallways in my wheelchair. The huge smile on my face let everyone know just how happy I was to be back at school. As Ryan pushed me through the crowds of students I was so excited to see people I had not seen since last spring. That first day we were late to nearly every class because we were only able to move a few feet before someone would stop and want to talk to us. Teachers came out of their classrooms to give me hugs and shake my hand and let me know how happy they were to have me back in school.

During ninth grade I was involved in nearly every extra-curricular club offered through the school. I was student council president, I was in the National Junior Honor Society, I was a peer mentor, and I was in the yearbook club. I loved being involved in my school and with my student groups.

When that first day of school ended I was exhausted, but I knew it was going to be a great year. After that first day of class my spirits were lifted, and I had a more positive mindset. Returning to school allowed me to surround myself with other kids and help bring some sense of normalcy back to my life. The focus of my time was shifted towards my friends and school, and away from worrying about my health.

The next day before I went to school, I had to go to Minneapolis for a checkup with the transplant team. I had an appointment that morning with Dr. Pritzker.

I entered Dr. Pritzkers office, and when he looked at me his entire face dropped. His expression changed and his smile slipped away. He drew in a deep breath, let out a long sigh and said, "Well, Nick, I hope you brought a bag with you, because by the looks of things, you will be staying in the hospital for a while."

The room spun by as I snapped my head around to look at Dr. Pritzker. I was having trouble fully understanding what he had just said. I cocked my head and looked at him, visibly confused. Dr. Pritzker approached me and motioned for my parents and me to sit. He looked at my parents and said, "Mr. and Mrs. Zerwas, we believe Nick needs a heart transplant soon, and we no longer believe Nick is healthy enough to continue waiting for a transplant at home."

I was speechless as I watched Dr. Pritzker talk to my parents; I stared at him while he explained to my parents his concerns. He talked about some different IV medications they would use to strengthen my heart while I waited in the hospital. Dr. Prtizker explained to my parents that I would be placed in the cardiac intensive care unit at Abbott Northwestern Hospital while I waited for a transplant. He then turned to me and asked, "Nick, do you think can wait in the hospital? Will you be able to handle that?"

Without pausing to think I immediately replied, "I will do whatever I need to do."

"It won't be easy, Nick. You could spend a long time in there; we still don't know when you will get a heart," he said.

"Dr. Pritzker, I will wait as long as I need to. I can handle it," I reassured him.

"Nick, don't take this personally, but once you're in the hospital, you won't last a month," he tersely responded.

"No. I will do whatever it takes. As long as I continue to breathe, I will continue to fight. I will never give up." My eyes filled with tears, and my voice quieted as a lump began to grow in my throat.

"Okay. Well, let's do it then," Dr. Pritzker said, obviously surprised by my response. "Tomorrow morning you can check in at the admission desk of the hospital, and we will get you all settled in a room."

That car ride from Minneapolis to Elk River reminded me of the trip home nine months earlier when we first found out that I needed a heart transplant. I sat in the back seat, trying with every fiber of my being not to cry. My dad stared straight ahead through the windshield, hardly making a sound. My mom began calling my grandparents and every other relative she promised to call after the doctor's appointment. She tried desperately to cheer everyone else up as she told him or her I was going to be admitted to the hospital. She mentioned the IV heart medication I would be on and how it would actually help strengthen my heart. At the end of every conversation the person she called was thanking her for cheering them up.

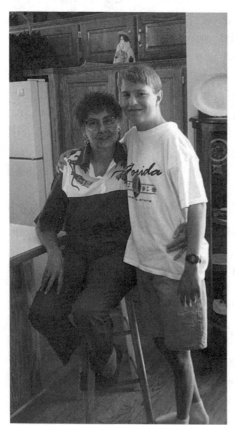

Nick and Grandma Palm, 1995

My dad and I went to the school that afternoon to meet with Mr. Gaarder, Mr. Weinman, and a few of my teachers in order to explain what was happening. Everyone at school was pretty shocked that I was going in the hospital the following day. They had all seen me one day earlier during the first day of the new school year, and determined that because I was smiling and I looked excited that I was feeling good. Mr. Conley agreed to be my home schoolteacher and to bring my homework down to the hospital every week. However, he was not comfortable with trying to teach me geometry. Doug Bloom, my geometry teacher, volunteered to drive to Minneapolis every week to help me with math. Mr. Bloom was a younger teacher, fairly new at the school, and I didn't know him that well. He was a young, single man with no children of his own, and he volunteered time out of his evenings to tutor a student he had only known for a little over a year.

The last evening I was home my mom and I packed some items from my bedroom to bring to the hospital. We packed books, videos, video games, and even my home computer. Not wanting to be stuck in hospital gowns and PJs everyday, nearly all of my clothes were packed in suitcases.

I fell asleep surprisingly quickly considering it was the last night I would be sleeping in my own bed for the foreseeable future. The next morning I woke up early, sat in my bed looking around my bedroom, and prayed that this wasn't going to be the last time I was here.

I was in high spirits as we entered the lobby of the hospital and found the registration desk. I laughed when the lady working the desk double-checked that I was really being admitted directly into the cardiac intensive care unit. I overheard her tell my parents that she had never heard of someone being admitted into the intensive care unit. I leaned forward and said, "Well, I heard they have bigger rooms, and better food down there."

Station 10, the cardiac intensive care unit at Abbott Northwestern Hospital, is a stark contrast to every other part of the hospital I have seen. Walking down the long hallway in the basement of the hospital towards the patient rooms reminded of a scene out of One Flew Over The Coocoo's Nest; there was no color or anything visually appealing. In order to get to the patient rooms you have to walk through the intensive care

.F.W. doles out cash to winners

Zerwas, Leonard, Keifenheim win top essay honors

A trio of Elk River High School students were honored last Tuesday at a V.F.W. meeting for their award-winning essays.

Nick Zerwas took first in the local installment of the 51st annual Voice of Democracy audio essay contest, while Emily Keifenheim took second and Jed Leonard took third. All three received cash prizes.

The local contest was sponsored by the Elk River-Rogers V.F.W. Post 5518 and its Ladies Auxiliary. It also sponsored a local contest in St. Francis for the first time. The theme of this year's contest was "My Voice in Our Democracy."

Zerwas and Leonard read their essays to veterans, ladies auxiliary members and family members at the ceremony. Keifenheim could not attend the ceremony, so she will read hers later.

Keifenheim

Leonard

'My Voice in Our Democracy'

Every day I find comfort in the fact that I am a United States citizen. My voice in our democracy, although quiet and raspy, damaged from five open heart surgeries, is just as highly regarded as the voice that booms out over all others. In a Democratic society like the United States, everyone has an equal voice in the direction their country is moving.

Over the last few years as I have gotten older, I have had more conversations with my grandmother, who was a teenager in World War II Germany. She tells stories of how she and other kids were forced to wear Nazi uniforms to a school that trained them on how to be future leaders of Europe dominated by Germany. And how the majority of the German citizens did not support, and wanted nothing to do with World War II, but were forced to ration their food and put the country before themselves. They had no say in the direction of their lives, or the direction of their country was traveling in, even when it was a matter of life and death. She has also told of the terrible conditions of human rights in Germany at the time. How people could not voice their opinions, or oppose in any way the tyranny they were living under, without facing death, or imprisonment. Also how the government decided who was fit to live, or who was too weak, or differ-

ent, and should die. If I had lived in World War II Germany, there was no way I would have received any medical treatment to keep me alive. Physically along with mentally handicapped people were shipped off to a slow death of starvation, or hypothermia in a concentration camp. Thousands of good capable people's voices in their democracy was stripped away from them, and then they were murdered. Just because people could not walk, or weren't as intelligent as the government believed

they should have been, they were seen as a burden on society, and they were killed.

I use a wheelchair to get around school because of my heart condition, but I feel that my voice in our democracy is just as important as a person that can run a marathon. In the United States all of its citizens have an important role to fill. Not just during an election year, but also writing your elected officials your ideas. After all, you are the ones that gave them their job. Shouldn't you now tell them what to do? Remember that in a democracy the voting major-

ity holds all the power to elect officials' ideas we like and vote out those who don't work for the country's best interest. For those teens that say that they have no voice because they can't vote, I say look around at what has been accomplished by people our age. In my hometown a walking bridge will be erected where a boy was hit by a car, after a petition started by teens was signed by over 7,000 people. Just because you can't vote doesn't mean your voice in our democracy should be muffled. I am confident in the fact that I do have a voice in our democracy, even if sometimes people have to listen harder to hear it.

— Nick Zerwas

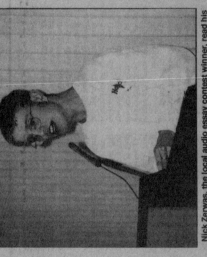

Nick Zerwas, the local audio essay contest winner, read his winning essay to a crowd at last week's V.F.W. meeting.

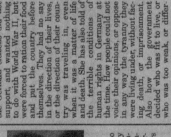

Star News article about Nick's first-place win in essay contest, "My Voice in Our Democracy"

waiting room, which is about as uplifting as attending a wake. Then as you enter the cardiac intensive care unit, you hear it. The beeping and chirping of heart monitors and the whooshing of ventilators. The constant bustle of the ICU is enough to make you exhausted just watching it.

We were met by a group of nurses who immediately showed us around. It wasn't long before I was settled into my room, Suite 6A. My hospital room was much larger than a standard hospital room. The nurses explained the room was originally used for patients on the Jarvic artificial heart, the first artificial heart in the United States. A large section of the room was now empty that used to be home to the large mainframe computer that ran the Jarvic artificial heart.

After the nurses got me settled into my room, and had started an IV, and had hooked up an EKG heart monitor, I began unpacking my things. It wasn't long until my computer was set up in the corner of the room and my walls were covered with posters and pictures of friends and family.

Those first few days in the hospital were actually a lot of fun. The nurses occupied my time by telling stories and bringing me around the hospital to see different things. Most of their patients were elderly people recovering from heart surgery. They loved entertaining me with pizza parties and practical jokes. I felt like part of the team, always sitting at the nurses' station and visiting with so many brilliant surgeons. I told my nurses things I was afraid to tell my parents—they always listened and cared.

Arrangements were made so I could go to the roof of the hospital and get a tour of the Life Link helicopter. A heart surgeon at the hospital allowed me to observe an open heart surgery. For the first time I was able to fully appreciate the atmosphere of a cardiac surgery. I was surprised by the amount of conversation that took place, but I was still impressed with the attention to detail and concentration on everyone's part.

I was surprised by the number of visitors I had in the hospital. During the first few days nearly all of my friends and family came to visit. Both of my grandparents, and all of my aunts and uncles, came to visit me. Dozens of friends from my neighborhood and VandenBerge Junior High came to visit along with their parents. Large groups would gather around my bed, and I would try to entertain them by recounting funny stories from the previous day. We would be talking loud and laughing in my room, and my nurse would have to close both doors to my room to try to keep the noise from bothering the other patients and families. I would laugh at some joke, and try to hush the room, so we didn't get any complaints from others in the unit. After the large groups of people left, my room would be eerily silent, and I couldn't wait for the next visitors to come.

A group of people from the Elk River Police Department, along with a few of my dad's cousins, worked together in order to plan one of the largest fundraisers in Elk River. Understanding the looming stress my extended hospitalization was putting on my parents, they decided it was necessary to raise money to help out my family. They knew my mom had taken a leave of absence from her job, and my dad's now daily commute to Minneapolis was going to be a tremendous hardship.

They were able to organize a fundraiser that included a dinner, dance, silent auction, and live auction. Nearly every business in Elk River donated money, their services, or products for the event. The Elk River Star News ran several stories and ads for the event to spread awareness throughout the community.

Although I wanted to attend the dance in the worst way, the doctors determined at that point I was just much too ill to leave the hospital. A capacity crowd filled the local VFW legion where the event was held, and the money raised was far beyond anyone's expectations.

My hospitalization was obviously an adjustment for my parents and their schedules. My mom, for all practical purposes, moved into the hospital along with me. Every night she would unfold a small cot in the corner of my hospital room and make her bed. She slept in the hospital room with me every weeknight, and joined my father in the hotel connected to the hospital on weekends. My dad was able to modify his schedule in order to spend more time at the hospital with us.

My grandma and grandpa came every other day. We played cribbage and spent hours together just talking.

During the week my dad, who was the police chief in Elk River, would arrive to work at the police department by 8:00 A.M. and attend to the pressing issues of the morning. Meetings that needed to occur were generally scheduled in the morning hours. By afternoon he had gathered the paperwork he needed to read through and begun the hour drive to Abbott Northwestern Hospital. In the corner of my hospital room my dad created a workspace with a small desk and a phone, and he worked out of my hospital room most afternoons. He would return phone calls to people in Elk River, and read through his officer's reports from previous shifts. He conducted most of his work as police chief from a cramped table in the corner of his son's hospital room. My dad would stay with my mom and me usually until around 9:00 or 10:00 P.M. He would then drive back to Elk River, go to sleep, and wake up the next morning to do it all over again. Then, on the weekends, he would stay with my mom in a hospital hotel room and spend the weekends with us at the hospital.

Mr. Conley and Mr. Bloom each came down to the hospital once a week to go over assignments from school. Mr. Bloom and I would work on my geometry assignments from his class. Mr. Bloom would come every week with a large pizza and some pop. He would review all of my homework assignments from the previous week, and he would answer any questions I had. Then he would explain the new assignments, and we would go over some example problems. It never failed that at some point I would become discouraged and say, "Bloom, this is stupid! Why do I even have to do this? Geometry is so pointless; I will never need to know this stuff."

Mr. Bloom would always reply, "Zerwas, dude, it's not that hard, and you do need to learn this because you need to pass my class." Then we would laugh, take a break, have another slice of pizza, and do some more sample problems.

When Mr. Conley would come down to the hospital, he would bring my assignments from the rest of my classes. He would very quickly and briefly explain what each teacher had asked him to tell me. Then he would give me a VCR tape to watch every week. The VCR tape was recorded each week by a different group of students that Mr. Conley had sent around the school to record different things. The tapes would usually have little messages recorded by students wishing me well, or just random video of students being silly. The weekly tapes helped keep me in touch with the students, and always helped brighten my day. Mr. Conley would also bring posters signed by students and staff. It wasn't long before large, colorful posters with hundreds of signatures from the people at VandenBerge Junior High covered every open space of wall in my room.

Karin visited me for the first time in the hospital after my first week. Her mom drove her down to Minneapolis so she could see me. When Karin was visiting me in the hospital, it was the first time since we started dating that we didn't have much to talk about. She looked upset when she saw me, and was unusually quiet during our whole visit. I kept telling her that I felt fine and I was doing great, but she knew better. After just a few uncomfortable visits to the hospital, that almost always ended with her being visibly upset when it was time for her to leave, I called Karin and asked her not to come down and visit anymore. I explained that it was just too difficult for me to see her upset. I apologized for the trouble I had caused for her and I hung up the phone.

The days after Karin and I stopped dating I sat in my hospital room bummed out. I deeply regretted hurting her feelings, and I resented being stuck in the hospital. I became restless, and I soon yearned to be back in Elk River with my friends in school and with my family at home.

Those feelings temporarily left one morning in early October. That morning I woke up early as a nurse entered my hospital room to draw blood. She drew blood out of my PIC line in my arm and told me to go back to sleep. When I asked what the blood was being drawn for, she gave a reason that didn't make much sense to me. I shrugged off the early morning incident, rolled over, and fell asleep. A few hours later I was awakened again, this time by my brother David walking into my room.

Confused, I looked at David and then at my clock, and realized it was only 5:00 A.M. My brother had a bewildered look on his face and asked me, "Nick, what are you doing?"

"I am sleeping. What do you want? What are you doing here?" I asked slightly aggravated, as I was not yet awake.

"I, uh, I just came by to say hi," he said, looking confused as he glanced around the room.

"What are you doing here? Why are you here so early?" I asked as I sat up in bed.

"Nick, I don't know why I am here. Mom and Dad called me at school and told me to get over here as fast as I could," he explained.

"Well, this is weird. I don't have a clue to what is going on around here. First I get woken up to get blood drawn, then you show up at 5:00 in the morning." My voice trailed off as my mind raced. "Wait! Dave!" I said raising my voice. "What if it's a match?" I asked.

I pressed my call button to call the nurse into my room. She looked a little confused as she came in. "A little early for visitors, isn't it?" she asked my brother.

David looked down and said, "My parents asked me to come over here."

"Okay, what's up?" I asked. "First, you come in and draw blood in the middle of the night, and then my parents tell David to come over here at 5:00 A.M. Something is going on."

"Nick, I already told you what the blood was for, and I don't know why your brother is here," she said with a large smile on her face.

"Just tell me if it is a heart. Did they find me a heart?" My voiced rose with excitement as I asked the question.

"Nick, I am sorry, but I can't be the person to tell you. So, I have to go back outside to the nurses' station. Your parents will be here shortly," she said as she left the room.

David sat in a chair in the recliner of my room and stared across the room at me. I looked back at him and said, "Well, looks like this is going to be a busy day."

Just then the telephone rang in my room. "Hello," I said, picking up the phone.

"Hi, Nick, it's Mom. Dad and I are on our way. We will be there in a little bit," she shouted into the phone.

"Hi, Mom, how are you…"

"Has Dr. Pritzker been in to see you yet? What did he say? Have they told you what time people should be there by, to see you before you go in?" she said, still talking very loudly.

"No, no, and no. Mom, nobody here has told me anything. All I know is David showed up and …"

"Oh, okay, David is there…good. Well, okay, Honey, sounds good. We will be there in a little bit."

"Hey, Mom," I said, trying to get her attention.

"What, Nick?" she asked.

"You picked a bad night to go home and clean the house," I said, laughing.

"We are almost there. We gotta go. Bye!" she said as she hung up the phone.

"Well, Dave, they are going nuts," I said, shaking my head.

David and I watched some television while we waited for my parents to arrive. After a few minutes, Dr. Pritzker walked into my room, looked at my brother, shook his head, and said, "Well, I see they still can't keep a secret down here if their life depended on it."

I smiled broadly, looked at Dr. Pritzker and said, "So, it's true. They found a match?"

"Well, everything looks good. They are going to run one last test to check for antibody reactions, but it is the right size and blood type. Everything should work out just fine," Dr. Pritzker said very proudly.

"Okay, what should I do until we know for sure?" I asked.

"Sit back and relax. It will be a long morning, so just relax," he said, patting me on the back.

A few minutes after Dr. Prtizker confirmed what was going on and left my room to do his morning rounds, my parents arrived. My dad gave me a large hug, patted me on the back, and sat down at the desk. He began making phone calls, working down our phone list, letting people know what was going on this morning.

My mom began grilling my brother and me about what Dr. Pritzker said when he was in my room. We told her that he said we were waiting for one last test, and that it would be a long morning. As my parents got settled in and worked on calling on more friends and family members, I lay down in bed and fell back asleep. I dozed on and off for a few hours, delaying the stress of being awake as long as possible. Finally, when I could no longer lie still, I decided to get up.

The hospital room was buzzing with quiet whispers as my brothers visited and joked; my mom talked nervously to a few nurses. Everyone was so preoccupied with the good news of the morning that hardly anyone noticed I was awake. When my mom finally glanced over at my hospital bed she smiled broadly and said, "Good morning, sleepy head! I thought you were going to sleep all day long."

"No," I quietly replied, glancing around the room and waving at my brothers. "Where is Dad?"

"Dad is in the waiting room," she said.

"Oh. Why is he sitting out there by himself?" I asked, a little confused.

My mom smiled and shook her head, "Nick, he isn't by himself, he is out there with everyone who is waiting."

"Who is all out there waiting?" I pressed.

"Everyone who found out about the heart. All of your aunts and uncles, friends from school. Everyone!" she continued. "Dr. Pritzker said everything looks good, and soon we will get the rest of the test results back."

I nodded my head in understanding and glanced up at the clock. The pit in my stomach grew as I realized the surgery would be coming very soon. A moment later my nurse came into the room and explained that it was time to prep for the surgery. She helped me to the bathroom, where she unwrapped the special surgical soap and explained the importance of scrubbing my chest very thoroughly. I climbed into the hot shower and began slowly and methodically scrubbing my chest, replicating what the nurse had instructed. The combination of the steam from the shower and me standing up for a few minutes soon made me feel light headed. As I sat in the chair mounted in the handicapped shower stall, I began to imagine life after the transplant. First I thought of the little things, like being able to stand in the shower, and being able to walk up a flight of stairs. Then I began to imagine things I never really thought were possible before, like graduating from high school, and then college. Maybe one day even having a wife and family of my own. The lump in my throat and tears running down my cheeks, along with the shower water, pulled me back into reality. I coughed and cleared my throat, shut off the water in the shower, and asked my nurse if she would help me get out.

After scrubbing for surgery, I returned to my hospital bed to get the final word from Dr. Pritzker that the surgery was a go. The last few moments I visited with my brothers, my mom and dad. We laughed and joked and hugged and cried. We coped with the stress the way we had so many times before when we all came together as a family.

Soon Dr. Prtizker came into the room and sat in the chair across from my bed. When I looked into his eyes I was immediately crushed, because I knew what was coming next.

"Tom, Chris, Nick…" he began, glancing around the room and then down at the floor. "The final tests are in…and…Nick, I'm sorry…but this heart just isn't going to work. It's not a match," he choked out, his eyes glossy as he looked at me for forgiveness.

"What!? No! How…how is it not a match?" my mom began asking. "What's wrong? Why didn't this match?" she continued.

My dad sat motionless in his chair, and finally just dropped his head down to his chest and began weeping. My brothers, who were sitting next to each other, broke down, too.

"Nick," Dr. Pritzker continued, "the good news out of all of this is that Leonard, the sixty-five-year-old patient down the hall, is going to be getting the heart. Don't worry, we will get you one."

I nodded my head and lay down in bed. As I lay in bed I began to feel stupid. Stupid for getting excited, stupid for thinking about going to college, stupid for thinking all along that everything was going to be all right.

As I fell asleep my dad went into the waiting room to tell the rest of the family and all of my friends that I would not be getting a heart transplant today, but thanks anyway for coming down. The waiting room was filled with shock and disappointment, and my dad was there to comfort those who had come down to support us.

Watching My Funeral
11

The days following the rejection of that first cross-matched heart were very difficult. That night, the dreams began coming to me in my sleep. The dreams were so terrifying that I soon avoided sleeping at night. I began dreaming about death and dying. Every dream, no matter how innocent it began, ended with me sitting at a funeral in the midst of a crowd, looking at my body in the casket.

I stayed in bed all day long, and I instructed the nurses not to allow visitors. During these days I was very selfish, and I wouldn't even get out of bed for my parents. I slept almost all day, and cried almost all through the night, only telling my primary nurses about my fears. As usual, I protected my family as much as I could by not telling them about the dreams.

Momentarily I had, without a doubt, given up. I had resigned, resigned not to fight, and resigned to die. I had accepted that it was over, and that I was going to die soon. This, however, didn't last long. If one thing was for sure, my mom did not raise a quitter.

"Nicholas! Get up!" my mom yelled.

I pulled the covers off my face and looked around my hospital room. Startled, I tried to figure out what was going on. My mom was standing next to me, yelling at me to get out of bed. The room was dark and otherwise quiet. She began pulling my covers back as she kept yelling at me to get up. Confused from just waking up, I followed her commands. She lifted me up and sat me up in bed. I looked across at her and I realized just how upset she was.

"Nick!" she said through her tears, "You need to get up. You can't do this to yourself. Nick, you have to stay positive, we have to stay positive." I nodded my head in agreement, and she continued, "Nick, I can't make it through this without you, and you can't make it through this on your own. None of us can handle this alone. We need to support each other, we all need everyone's support."

"I know...I know," I said quietly as I leaned forward and hugged my mom. "I'm sorry, I just didn't think I could do it. I didn't think I could handle not getting that heart. I was just so devastated I didn't know what to do. I know I need to talk to you guys, but it's so hard. I just feel so sad, and I don't want to be this sad anymore." I continued crying harder now, "All I want is to know that everything will work out. That no matter what we have to go through, and no matter how long it takes, that everything will be okay."

"I know, I know, Sweetie, but you know we can't possibly know that. All we can do is live everyday, and you need to start doing that again. You have been holed up here in your room for a week, and that's not healthy. You can't just lie here; while you are here, you have to live here," she said.

"You're right, I know I have to get up. Mom, thanks for picking me up, and kicking my butt a little. I needed that," I joked.

After that intervention by mom I was able to pull myself, and my spirits, up. I still struggled with a lot of feelings and fears, especially at night. I was alone during the night; my nurse would check on me from time to time, but in all reality I was alone. It was at night when I was alone that I had time to think. Think about the future, think about being sick, and think about death. Every night I would try pushing all of those thoughts out of my head, and rest. As I drifted off to sleep every night those fears came creeping back. Several times a night I would wake up recalling with vivid details the dream of my funeral. Every night I watched from the last pew in the church a funeral ceremony. It wouldn't become apparent that I was at my own funeral until everyone filed past the casket, and it wasn't until then that I would realize it was me in the casket, and my funeral. I would watch my parents sob, and not be able to comfort them. I could see my brothers unable to stand, but I couldn't help them. Every night I was forced to watch this scenario play out in my head, helpless to stop it.

As my spirits began to go back up the days went by quicker. Soon the visitors that avoided the hospital for a while after the heart didn't match resumed visiting. During the next month I fell into a routine of working on schoolwork, meeting with my teachers, and receiving visitors. The weekends were always packed, usually with large groups of friends and family making the trip into Minneapolis to come visit. We would visit, watch movies, and my friends would tell me all the latest news and gossip from school.

In late October Dr. Pritzker met with me and my family to discuss future options. He was concerned that I had spent too much time in the hospital and wanted to send me home for a while. The idea of being able to go home was both very exciting and very frightening. Over the course of the last few months I could tell I was feeling weaker, and my heart was not as strong as before I was admitted into the hospital. After that meeting with Dr. Pritzker, plans were made very quickly for me to be released from the hospital. Within a few days home healthcare nurses met with my parents and me to coordinate my care in Elk River.

I was released from Abbot Northwestern's Station 10 Cardiac Intensive Care Unit on October 31, 1995. I was so excited to be home, handing out the Halloween candy to the trick-or-treaters all night long. My dad and I took a quick break from answering the door that evening to drive a few blocks to Mrs. Erickson's house. I had been trick-or-treating at her house for several years in a row, and she always handed the jumbo-sized candy bars. I knocked on her front door, and I waited and smiled. Mrs. Erickson answered the door and immediately started screaming. I told her I would be out of the hospital for a while, and I would be coming back to her English class at VandenBerge Junior High next week. When she heard that, she immediately threw her arms around me and began to cry. I was so glad to be out of the hospital.

The next week I went back to school part-time; I attended the first three classes of the day a few times a week. I still did the majority of my coursework with my geometry teacher, Mr. Bloom, who was still homeschooling me, but it was still good to be back in class. I was surrounded by my friends and people who supported me the whole time I was away, and that was a tremendous boost to my spirits. Being at school every morning and surrounded by people and activity made the time pass by very fast.

Staying at home was difficult, however. My body was very rundown, and my medications were constantly being changed. I began having problems with retaining fluid, which made my heart have to work harder to pump the blood through my body. Almost on a weekly basis I was admitted to the hospital to be put on IV diuretics to force my body to void off the excess fluid. This routine became difficult and tedious, but it allowed me to stay at home.

I had frequent appointments with Dr. Pritzker and the rest of the transplant doctors while I was out of the hospital. During one of the visits Dr. Pritzker explained his concerns and strategies for finding me a donor heart.

"Nick, we talked before about your high antibody level possibly making it more difficult to find you a donor heart that would match," he began. "This concern has proven itself true; your body has rejected the few organs we have cross-matched you with. My fear is that if we leave things the way they are we will not find a heart that will be compatible with your body."

"Does that mean I won't be able to get a heart transplant?" I interjected.

"Well…" Dr. Pritzker continued, "what it means is that we will have to take more proactive steps in order to find you a matching organ."

"Proactive steps? Is it really legal to roam the streets looking for a donor?" I asked with a smile.

"That's not exactly what I meant by proactive," Dr. Pritzker laughed. "What we want to do," he continued, "is reduce the antibody level in your body by reducing your immune system. By lowering your immune system before surgery we should be able to find a matching heart, allow that heart to get accustomed to your body, and then gradually bring your immune system back up."

"How do you lower Nick's immune system in the first place?" my mom asked.

"What prevents you from lowering his immune system too low, and having Nick develop an infection?" my dad asked.

"Nick's immune system would be lowered using plasmaphoresis and Cytoxin. Basically, a machine will remove blood from Nick, that blood will be spun at high speeds, and the immune system cells will be removed from the blood. That blood would then be reintroduced into Nick," Dr. Pritzker explained.

"And the Cytoxin?" I asked apprehensively. "I try to shy away from anything with the word 'toxin' in the title—it's bad for my diet," I said joking.

"Cytoxin is a chemotherapy drug used for cancer patients. Cytoxin kills cells that replicate quickly, usually tumor cells, but also immune cells," Dr. Pritzker explained.

"And hair follicles," I asserted.

"What was that?" Dr. Pritzker asked.

"And hair follicles. Cells that replicate quickly and are killed by chemotherapy drugs; tumor cells, immune cells, and hair follicles," I repeated.

"Yes, you are right. However, the dose of Cytoxin given to you will be much lower, and probably not result in your hair falling out," he explained. "Tom, Chris, Nick, I want you to know we have been discussing this a great deal while Nick has been at home the last several weeks, and there really is no other viable alternative. It is time to take drastic measures in order to find a donor heart that will match Nick."

Dr. Pritzker explained that all of the details of the new procedures were being worked out and that I would be readmitted to Abbott Northwestern Hospital a few weeks after the holidays. My parents and I believed this would be my only hope to receive a heart transplant, and we were anxious to begin.

That year, both my birthday in mid December and Christmas passed with a sense of uneasiness. I turned fifteen years old, and my parents gave me an old car for my birthday, so I could learn to drive once I got better. I remember sitting in that car for the first time that day wondering if I would ever get my license. I remember hardly being able to imagine living through another year like the one that was quickly coming to an end.

I was able to see both sides of my extended family over Christmas, something I had enjoyed very much. They had all come down to visit me in the hospital at one time or another, but it was very special to be surrounded by loved ones and family at Christmas.

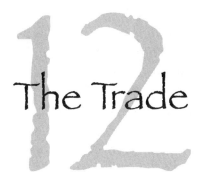

The Trade

The weeks following Christmas I quickly got my affairs in order at school and prepared to go back into the hospital. The morning I checked back into Station 10 at Abbott Northwestern Hospital, a large group of nurses were waiting in my hospital room to welcome me back. They greeted us with hugs, and told me how glad they were to be able to take care of me again.

The first night back in the hospital I stayed awake most of the night visiting with my nurses. We talked about the new plasmaphoresis and Cytoxin I would be undergoing beginning the following day. They wished me luck, and told me everything was going to be okay.

Early the next morning I was brought into surgery where a cardiac surgeon was going to place a catheter through my chest wall into the top of my heart. I was joking around and laughing with the surgical staff as I was wheeled into the operating room. I transferred beds on to the operating room table, told a few final jokes, and laid my head back. As I lay down I said to the operating room staff, "Well, goodnight everyone!"

The surgeon bent way down in front of my face and said, "Nick, somebody talked to you about this surgery, right?"

I looked up at the surgeon, smiled and said, "Yeah, its just a tube through my chest into my heart. I have had way more complicated surgeries—you'll do fine."

"No, Nick. What I meant is, I was wondering if someone met with you this morning to tell you we wouldn't be putting you to sleep for this operation."

"Why not? Why would you keep me awake while you dig through my chest wall?" I asked, the anxiety now noticeable in my voice.

"Nick, if we put you to sleep without giving you a new heart, we don't think you would wake up," the surgeon said very casually.

"Nick, don't worry about a thing. You may be awake, but I'll make sure you just don't give a damn," the anesthesiologist said.

Shortly after that I drifted off into a layer of consciousness somewhere between totally asleep and somewhat awake. I was totally aware of my surroundings, but the surgeon tugging and cutting at my chest just did not bother me in the slightest bit.

Later that afternoon while I was still recovering from the placement of the catheter for the plasmaphoresis, I actually began my first round of the plasmaphoresis. At this time I also took the first of the fluorescent green Cytoxin pills. I lay in my hospital room with my parents sitting next to me while this large machine rumbled to my side. Visible in the "in and out" tubes going to the machine was a constant supply of my blood being sucked into the machine, and then fed back into me.

Time once again slowed down dramatically now that I was back in the hospital. The few hours a day during the plasmaphoresis seemed to stretch on for days by themselves. The combination of plasmaphoresis and the chemotherapy quickly made me feel even more tired. Within a few weeks after beginning the chemotherapy and the plasmaphoresis, my appetite dropped off and I was unable to eat.

One morning, several weeks after being readmitted into the hospital, I felt sick to my stomach when I woke up. I tried to eat a little of my breakfast, hoping a piece of toast would settle my upset stomach. Later that morning I got sick and vomited. Throwing up had really tired me out, so I went back to sleep. A while later I woke up again with an upset stomach and threw up once again. That first day that I got sick from the chemotherapy I threw up over twenty-five times. From that point on I was sick almost constantly. I woke up vomiting and I fell asleep vomiting. The smell or the mere mention of food made my stomach turn. I lost thirty pounds almost immediately. I had absolutely no appetite, and on the few occasions I did get some food down, it would almost certainly come right back up.

While I was waiting for a heart at Abbott, it wasn't long before my parents and I began hearing about a twenty-two-year-old woman who was in critical condition across the street at Minneapolis Children's Hospital. It seems Molly went in to Minneapolis Children's for a redo of her Fontan heart surgery. During the middle of her open heart surgery, Molly's heart went into cardiac arrest and stopped. The doctors at Children's Hospital worked tirelessly to revive her heart and keep her alive. They succeeded in restarting Molly's heart, and she lived. Now Molly was in the Intensive Care Unit at Minneapolis Children's on a respirator, with only a few days to live.

When I heard about Molly with so little time left to live, I looked at my parents and said, "I have to do something. I have to save her."

I met with the coordinator of the transplant program, Mary O'Kane, along with Dr. Pritzker. I told them I wanted Molly to take my spot on the transplant list. Both Mary O'Kane and Dr. Pritzker insisted that would not be possible; the transplant program did not work that way. They explained that I had been in the Intensive Care Unit much longer than anyone else, and that I could not trade my number one spot on the list for her number two spot. I told them I understood that we couldn't swap spots. I then asked Mary to pull me off the transplant list until the girl in the hospital across the street either received a new heart or died. I told her I would never be able to live with myself if I got a donated heart before someone who was not even healthy enough to breathe on her own. In total disbelief they both left the room. Later that day I was informed by my nurse that I had been pulled from the transplant list.

Two days after my name was removed from the top of the waiting list we got word that a donor was found, and the heart would be going to the girl in the hospital across the street. Later that evening I watched as Molly was wheeled into her intensive care room at Abbott Northwestern Hospital to recover from her heart transplant. The following day I was informed by the transplant coordinator, May O'Kane, that my name was placed back on the heart transplant waiting list.

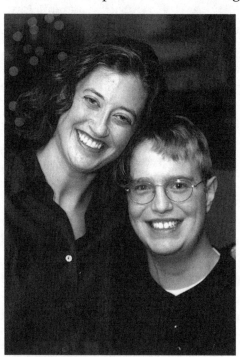

Nick and Molly Friedman, 1997
In the words of Molly, "I am the beneficiary of this man's heroic decision to save another's life while waiting for his own chance."

After Molly had recovered from her transplant and had left the Intensive Care Unit, the excitement in Station 10 dropped off. The days grew long and boring for me. The plasmaphoresis and the Cytoxin had lowered my immune system, so I was now in an isolated room. The double doors leading to my hospital room were kept closed, and visitors to my room had to wash their hands before entering. As I was an avid fan of the television sitcom Seinfeld, I would often joke about being the obnoxious "Bubble Boy" character. My mom and I would laugh until we cried as we played out scenes from the show. In that episode the sick kid, "Bubble Boy," exemplified how I was feeling at the time. Everyone in Bubble Boy's hometown knew of him and his illness, but in the show Bubble Boy is shown with only his family around him. Even though I wasn't physically inside a bubble, at this point I definitely felt very isolated from everyone.

I was still having difficulty eating any sizeable meals, and the pace of my vomiting really hadn't slowed down at all. I was still throwing up several times, which added to my discomfort. My weight loss was becoming very noticeable, and Dr. Pritzker scheduled dieticians to visit me and design meals high in calories. My parents did their best to try to find food that I would eat. They would bring me fast food, ribs, steak, shrimp, basically anything I said I would eat. Soon nothing sounded good to me, and I was going whole days with hardly eating any food.

My cardiologists were convinced my heart failure was so advanced that my central nervous system was shutting down my digestive system to conserve energy. Meanwhile, the psychologist that had begun seeing me was convinced that my lack of appetite was actually me displaying symptoms of anorexia. He was positive that I wasn't eating because the only thing I had control over in my life at that time was what food I put into my body.

When I was that sick I would have eaten more if I could have. The chemotherapy drugs had made me so weak and so sick that even the mention of food made my stomach turn. My mom would talk about one of my favorite foods to try to peak my interest. As she would talk about how good it would taste I would grab my bucket and begin to vomit. I was unable to associate anything positive with food while I was getting sick to my stomach so frequently.

After several month of undergoing the plasmaphoresis every other day, and taking the Cytoxin every morning, Dr. Pritzker told my parents and me that he would like to have a care meeting with several of the nurses, doctors, and our family. A few days later my brothers were at the hospital along with my parents and me to meet with the transplant team. Dr. Pritzker recapped my history since I began waiting in the hospital for a transplant to get everyone caught up.

"Nick was admitted to Station 10 in September of last year following a period of rapid decline in his cardiac output and function. Since being admitted to Station 10 Nick has been treated with IV drips to increase his cardiac output, and his heart rate and rhythm have been monitored constantly. Last fall it became apparent that Nick's high HLA antibody profile level was causing a greater degree of difficulty in finding a compatible donor organ then previously anticipated. Nick was discharged for a period of several months this winter in order to further develop a new plan. At that time the idea of immuno plasmaphoresis, along with a treatment of Cytoxin, was agreed upon as the best alternate way to introduce a donor heart into Nick's heightened immune system."

I looked around the room while Dr. Pritzker spoke, and all of the other doctors and nurses shook their heads in agreement with him. To my left, my parents sat next to each other holding hands tightly, hanging on to the doctor's every word.

"Now, Nick's antibody level before the plasmaphoresis and Cytoxin was at fifty-eight percent," Dr. Pritzker continued, "meaning Nick would reject fifty-eight percent of O-blood type donor hearts that a normal patient would not have a problem with. Recently, blood was drawn to check the new HLA antibody level after the immune system was lowered by the plasmaphoresis and the Cytoxin."

Dr. Pritzker breathed in deeply through his mouth, looked slowly around the room, then lowered his head and continued. "These recent antibody tests show a surprising result. Nick's HLA antibody profile went from fifty-eight to ninety-eight percent, meaning Nick would reject ninety-eight percent of all O-blood type hearts."

My face fell into my hands and I leaned over on my dad. I buried my face into his chest, and for the first time I realized I was never going to get a heart transplant. My dad put his arms around me, squeezed me tight, and held me there. I could hear my brothers crying on my right, and I could hear my mom crying and whispering to my dad, but I couldn't understand what was being said.

Dr. Pritzker began speaking once again, "Tom, Chris, and Nick, we brought everyone together today because it is time to decide what to do next."

"Well, if the damn Cytoxin isn't working, stop that first thing. I am tired of feeling so miserable, and if it's not even making a difference..." I stopped speaking, only because I could tell I was about to start crying again.

"Yes, definitely, we are going to halt the plasmaphoresis and the Cytoxin. As for your nausea, that may continue for a while after the Cytoxin is stopped while that drug works its way out of your system. My question, as far as what's next, has more to do with what your wishes are, Nick. If your heart begins to fail more, would you like to be put on a pump to help pump the blood for your heart? Normally, a pump like this would act as a bridge for someone who is waiting for a heart transplant," Dr. Pritzker explained.

"But for me this pump would be what?" I interrupted.

"It would be a bridge to nowhere. Nick, you are never going to get a heart transplant. If this pump is implanted in your chest, you will be in intensive care for the rest of your life, pulling this machine behind you down the hallway. You will be alive, but you will never be healthy enough to go home," he explained.

"It sounds like you think this would be a bad idea. Are you not recommending we try this?" my mom asked.

"It's an option, but it is not one I would recommend. It would be a dead-end road," Dr. Prtizker said very matter-of-factly.

"Would I be able to talk?" I asked.

"What?" Dr. Pritzker asked with a smug look on his face.

"Would I be able to talk on this pump? Would I be able to think? Would I be able to communicate?" I asked, growing more upset.

"Of course you would be able to talk and think," he replied.

"Then how can I say no? How can I decide that I don't want to live any longer, missing the chance to tell my mom and dad that I love them, just because it would mean that I am stuck here. Trust me, I hate this place more than anyone here, but the alternative doesn't sound much better. If living the rest of my life here meant I could still tell my parents what they mean to me, then I guess I would stay here," I said, sobbing hard.

I stood up from the conference table, excused myself, and went back to my hospital room. I sat on my hospital bed, still shocked that I would no longer be waiting for a heart transplant. My dad came into the room a few minutes after me and sat on the edge of my bed. He grabbed my foot and squeezed. He looked at me and said, "You know, Bud, we are going to figure something out. It will all work out somehow."

Soon my brothers, my mom, and Dr. Pritzker all walked into my room. Dr. Pritzker looked at me from across the room and said, "Nick, I'm sorry, but you are not going to get a heart transplant. There is nothing else we can do to help you find a heart. You have around six months left to live. Nick, please go home, be with your family and make the most of what you have left."

"Okay," I said quietly, not even looking up at him.

All together I had been cross-matched seventeen times for a new heart. I met many friends who got new hearts at Abbott. I knew they had done their best, and I would be forever grateful for all they tried.

Arrangements were made with the home health care nurses, and I was released from Abbott Northwestern Hospital a few days later. As I left Station 10 that morning it was very different from when I left on Halloween. I was not excited to be leaving, and it was obvious my nurses didn't want me to leave either. The nurses who cared for me most often all huddled around me as I prepared to leave. They hugged me and held me close as they all wished me good luck.

When we arrived at home I was almost in a daze. I still couldn't believe I was no longer waiting for a transplant. My appetite still had not returned even though I had been off of the chemotherapy drugs for over a week. My energy level was very low, and I was surprised at the difficulty I was having at home. While I was in the hospital, the most I would do in a day is get cleaned up, and if I were feeling well, I would walk a little bit around the floor. Now that I was at home I realized just how limited I was. I found it difficult to get myself something to drink or to walk from my bedroom out into the living room.

After I was home for a few days I started going to school again at VandenBerge Junior High. My dad drove me to school in the morning for two class periods. I only had enough energy to go for those first two classes. Mid morning my dad would drive back up to the school, pick me up, and drive me home. Going back to school was very exciting; all of my friends were thrilled to see me. Just being around people my age every day really helped in bringing up my spirits.

My parents talked to the principal, Mr. Gaarder, and explained to him the news from the doctors. Mr. Gaarder let some of the staff know that I was no longer a candidate for a transplant. I would usually be very good at keeping myself together while I was at school, but several times I had teachers approach me while no students were around to tell me they had heard what the doctors had said. Those first few weeks back in class I found myself hugging a lot of my teachers, and telling them not to worry.

I always told people who talked to me about not getting a heart transplant "not to worry," that "everything was going to be okay." The truth was, I was sure that everything wasn't going to be fine. I was positive that in a few months I would be dead. Most of time during this period was consumed with thinking about death. Every moment I was alone I obsessed with planning my funeral. I picked out the songs that I wanted sung, I chose casket bearers, I selected who would speak about me, I even chose the route for the funeral procession to wind through Elk River on its way to St. Andrew's Cemetery. I constantly wrote and rewrote these plans down nearly every time I was by myself. Then I would cry; I would cry until I couldn't cry any longer, until the thought of crying anymore just hurt too much to bear. Then, every time, I would rip up the paper, ashamed at myself for thinking so negatively.

The last week of ninth grade was a surreal experience for me. All of my classmates were excited that summer was finally here. I was dreading summer break, because I knew I would probably never see most of my friends again. By this time most of my close friends started to realize I was not going to receive a heart transplant, and without a new heart I wasn't going to survive much longer.

The last day of school was hard from the very beginning of the day. My dad drove me to class that morning, and said it would be okay if I wanted to stay the whole day. I was very happy to be able to be there the entire time. Our yearbooks were handed out first thing that morning. Like most of the students in my class, I flipped through the yearbook to find pictures of me with my friends. As I casually flipped through the annual I noticed several of my classmates staring at me and whispering. My best friend, Ryan, was seated next to me, so I leaned over and asked him what was going on. Ryan opened his yearbook to the last page, and told me people were noticing the dedication.

The final page in my ninth grade yearbook is a picture of me seated in my wheelchair. The message underneath the photo explained that I was extremely ill, and at the time of publication I was still alive and waiting for a heart transplant. It was clear to me, and most of my friends who saw that dedication, that they believed I would not be alive by the time the yearbook was in print.

I lost my grandfathers both within a few months, both of lung cancer. I kept wondering if God took them so they would be there in heaven waiting for me. I knew I was going to do my best for my grandfathers, but I was scared.

Dedication

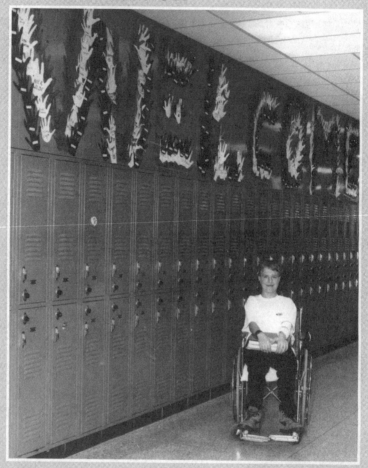

The members of the VandenBerge Jr. High School Yearbook Staff would like to dedicate the 1996 ANTLER to Nicholas Zerwas. At the time of this writing Nick is waiting for a heart donor and, when not at the hospital, has been busy here at school. Nick's courage and cheerful disposition has been an example to all of us and has made VandenBerge a better place because of his being here.

The above photo shows a part of a wall display of hand cut-outs which were placed in the hallway to welcome Nick back to school. Students from all grades helped produce this display by making signed hand forms of red, white and black paper.

Dr. Stone
And The Bovine Gift

A few weeks after school let out for the summer, I received a phone call from my original pediatric cardiologist, Dr. Stone. Dr. Stone explained that he had heard that I was no longer being considered for heart transplantation due to my high antibody level. Dr. Stone explained that he had been researching some alternate procedures that might be an option for me. Dr. Stone asked my parents to bring me in for an appointment. This phone call, and the news of hope, came as an unbelievable shock for me. I was very guarded about the whole matter, not wanting to get my hopes up.

The next week we went in to meet with Dr. Stone in his office. He explained again some of the ideas he had briefly mentioned over the phone. "Nick, I really don't think we can give up on your heart. The right-sided failure is pretty evident right now, but even still your cardiac output from the left side is remarkable. If we could tighten up that right atrium and allow the blood to pass straight through, rather than swirling around in the enlarged atrium, I believe the left side's function may be enough on its own."

"What would you do to the right atrium to allow the blood to flow directly through? How would you 'tighten' up the right atrium?" my mom asked, a hint of excitement in her voice.

"Well, that's what we need to decide on. There may be several ways to go about this procedure, but the most likely technique would be to remove most of the enlarged right atrium's outer wall. In its place a new passage would be constructed using bovine pericardium."

"Bovine pericardium? You mean you want to do a transplant with a cow?" I asked, half jokingly.

"Not exactly," Dr. Stone laughed. He continued, "What we would do is create a rigid passage for blood to flow through out of the sac that goes around a cow's heart. This would make the blood flow directly through the right side of your heart, not allowing the blood to swirl around. By decreasing the size of the tube the blood can flow through, the pressure is automatically increased. In theory, the output from the right side of your heart would increase, even though most of the muscle would be removed."

"This sounds new. Has it worked before?" my mom asked.

"This has never been tried in Minnesota before. They have had some success with procedures similar to this on the East coast," Dr. Stone said.

"Chances?...Um, do you know what the chances would be of a success?" I stammered.

"You know, that's a hard question to answer. There would be several complicating factors, including your previous surgeries and how sick you are before the surgery. The surgery is certainly risky, but if you do nothing, the odds are one hundred percent that you will be dead within a few months," he said solemnly.

"Well, I don't know about my parents, but my summer is pretty free, so I guess I'll do it," I said.

The night before the surgery my parents, my brother Tommy and his wife Karla, along with their daughter Makayla, my brother David, and I, all went out to dinner at the Mall of America. I ordered a rack of ribs and ate while I visited with my family. My parents were very quiet, which was normal for them before a surgery. Unfortunately, the side effects from the Cytoxin had still not totally passed, and I was not able to finish my dinner. My appetite was a little better then a few months earlier, but nowhere near where it had been before the chemotherapy. We drove to our hotel in Minneapolis and checked into our room. My mom was not feeling very well so she went up to the room to lie down. My dad and I sat in the hotel bar and talked for hours. I sipped on my cherry Coke and told him how hard it was for me to be in the hospital for so long. I explained how bad I felt for putting him and Mom through so much stress. Most of all, I thanked him. I told him how much it meant to me when he brought all of his work down to my hospital room and worked from there. I tried to explain to him how much having him and my mom as parents made me want to be a better person. At the end of the night, I gave my dad a hug, and we went up to our hotel to try to sleep.

The next morning we arrived at the hospital by 6:00 A.M. As we walked into the lobby, the walls were lined with family and friends who arrived early just to see me before I went into surgery. My grandma, along with aunts, uncles, cousins, and friends from school, were all there. After greeting everyone, I went back into the pre-op area and prepared for the surgery. After we met one last time with Dr. Stone and the surgeon, Dr. Nicoloff, the nurse gave me a Valium and told my parents I would be taken back into surgery in a few minutes. My brothers immediately sprung up from their chairs and came to the side of my hospital bed. Tommy laid his head down on my chest, nearly crushing me under his body. "I love you. I love you," he said through his sobs.

David lay across me from the other side of my bed. As he tried to speak he just cried louder and louder. He was never able to utter a single recognizable word. My parents stood behind David holding each other. My mom rubbed David's back trying to console him.

"Guys, I am going to be okay. Everything will be fine," I said strongly.

My mom leaned down by me and began to cry as I hugged her. She looked at me as if it was the last time she would ever see me again.

"Mom," I whispered to her. "Mom, don't be afraid. Everything will be fine. Today is just another day. If God decides my time is up today, then there is nothing we can do to change that. I really believe we are on Earth until our mission is complete. When we are done, we are done. It doesn't matter if we are having open heart surgery, or crossing the street. When our time is up, it is up. I don't think this surgery is anymore risky than the drive from the hotel over here this morning. If God believes my work here is done, trust me, it won't take open heart surgery to bring me to heaven. Today is no more risky than any other day. When my time is up it's up, and if it's not up yet, then a little surgery won't stop me."

She clung to my hospital gown and said, "That's the most brave, mature thing I have ever heard anyone say. I love you so much."

The anesthesiologist entered the room and announced it was time. I waved at everyone as he wheeled me out of the room and down the long hallway towards the operating room. When I was lying on the operating room table, the surgeon, Dr. Nicoloff, leaned down to say hi.

"Dr. Nicoloff, can I ask you a question?"

"Go ahead, Nick," he said while he was preparing for the surgery.

"Dr. Nicoloff, if I make it through this surgery, can I drive your Ferrari?" I asked with a broad smile.

"What, are you crazy?" he said. "Nick, I don't even let my wife drive that car."

"Okay," I said in a teasing voice.

"I will tell you what. When you are all healed, call me up, and I will have you over to the house and you can ride in whatever car you want," he said with a smile.

When I woke up in the Intensive Care Unit at Minneapolis Children's Hospital, I couldn't believe I had made it through the surgery. As the anesthesia began to wear off and I was able to think more clearly, I realized everything was going to be okay. My recovery after surgery was very quick. I was released from the hospital less then a week after the operation. I recovered from the surgery at home for the rest of the summer, and I was able to start school in the high school in September.

High School With A Different Stroke

"Nick, look at the pictures I found for your graduation open house," my mom said. "Oh, this was your first surgery," she said as she blinked away tears.

"It's okay, Mom, don't cry," I said.

"Did I tell you I made a deal with God the day of your first surgery? I know you're not supposed to, but I did. After I handed you over for surgery, we all went to the chapel. I told God if he wasn't going to let me keep you longer than seven years, that I would rather he took you that day, at three months old," she began.

"I looked at Tommy and David and knew how much I would love you every day. But, if I couldn't hear you say, 'I love you, Mommy,' and go to school, and do all the things I had been able to do with your brothers, then I asked God to take you that day. If you survived that first surgery, I told God I would take it as a message that he would let you stay with us for a long time," she said, wiping away her tears.

"I guess he was listening to you, Mom," I said as I gave her a big hug. "I remember the first day of high school; I never thought I would make it to high school."

The first day of tenth grade at Elk River High School was an unbelievable moment for me. I had been told so many times that I wouldn't live long enough to attend high school, it really felt like a miracle. I was so happy to be able to walk through the halls of the high school and no longer be in a wheelchair. After such a long and uncertain summer, it was also very comforting to be around my friends at school, and have the opportunity to make new friends in the high school.

The first few months of high school went by very quickly, and everything seemed normal. However, about halfway through my sophomore year I began to feel a little rundown. The first several weeks I thought I was feeling more tired then usual because of my hectic schedule, and possibly from fighting off a cold. As time continued to pass, and I did not start to feel any better, I realized something else might be wrong.

As my first year in the high school began to come to a close I started undergoing tests at the Children's Heart Clinic. Dr. Stone did not know why I was feeling so tired, but he was very concerned. The tests to determine what was causing my lack of energy continued on after school had let out for the summer. Soon my parents and I met with Dr. Stone to discuss the results of all the recent tests. He invited us into his office and began to explain what he had learned.

"We have been looking into Nick's complaints of feeling tired and decreased exercise tolerance for a while now. Nick did a stress test and walked on the treadmill while we monitored his heart. We then had Nick wear a 24-hour halter monitor to observe what his heart did throughout an average day. Finally, we did an angiogram, where we threaded a balloon up from Nick's leg into his heart. Once the balloon was positioned inside the heart, radioactive dye was released, and allowed us to get images of Nick's heart pumping blood," Dr. Stone explained.

My parents and I all nodded our heads in agreement, each one of us trying to anticipate what Dr. Stone would say next.

"All of these tests seem to indicate the same result. The bovine pericardium we used last summer to create a rigid narrow passage for the blood to travel through the right atrium has ballooned in size. In fact, the bovine pericardium is now as large as the failing right atrium muscle we removed in order to streamline the blood flow through the right side of the heart," Dr. Stone explained.

"So, we are right back in the same place as last summer. Nick's heart is enlarged, and it's failing," my mom said with a sense of disbelief.

Dr. Stone dropped his head slightly. "I am afraid so."

"Is there something else we can try? Another procedure? Something to take the place of the cow pericardium?" I pleaded.

"That's what we are hoping for. Dr. Nicoloff and I are looking around and talking to other people. He is very hopeful that he will be able to find something else to try, but it's going to take some time while we look into this. The good news is, physically you are in much better shape now compared to this time last year," he said, trying to lift my spirits. "Nick, Dr. Nicoloff and I are going to figure something out. Everything is going to be okay."

It was another long and quiet drove home to Elk River from Minneapolis. I sat in the back seat of the car in utter disbelief. I could not understand how I could be right back in the same position as one year earlier. I couldn't figure out how I could go through all that, and wind up in the exact same spot.

"This sucks!" I said from the backseat of my parent's truck.

"I know, Honey, this just isn't fair," my mom said, looking back at me.

"How could we end up right back in the same place? This is bullshit!" I shouted.

"Nicholas! Don't swear in front of your mother," my mom quietly scolded.

"Sorry," I said, feeling embarrassed. "You know, it just figures. I mean, everything was going so well—it just figures. It's like nothing can ever go smooth for us. Can I just have one school year where I don't miss at least one month for a surgery?" I continued.

My junior year of high school started soon after my doctor's appointment. Like so many recent years, I started the first day of eleventh grade in a wheelchair, being pushed to my classes by my best friend, Ryan, because I was unable to walk the distance between classrooms. The start of school that year was very depressing for me. I had really hoped I had left the days of being the sick kid, and the kid in the wheelchair, behind. This was the first time many of the people in the high school saw me so sick. Students and teachers were extremely nice to me, but I would have been much happier just being another healthy student in the crowd walking from class to class.

Later that fall my parents and I met again with Dr. Stone. I could tell when we walked into his office he was much happier now, compared to our earlier appointment. "Dr. Nicoloff and I have met several times and developed a plan to fix the blood flow on the right side of Nick's heart," he said, almost as soon as we walked into his office. "Dr. Nicoloff believes the best course of action would be to totally remove the bovine pericardium from Nick's heart. In its place we'll use a rigid piece of gortex to shape the conduit holding blood as it passes through the right side of the heart. This gortex conduit would be tougher than the bovine piece in place now. The increased rigidity of the material will help ensure that this new material will not be stretched by the high pressure, like both the heart muscle and the bovine pericardium tissue were stretched."

"You don't foresee any complications from trying to remove the bovine pericardium?" I asked.

"Well, this surgery will involve the same risks all of your recent heart surgeries have had. There is an increased risk of scar tissue, making it difficult to get at the heart. Once Dr.

Nicoloff has cut his way to the heart, he will have to cut the bovine pericardium tissue away. He then will take a flat piece of this fabric-like gortex material, and basically roll it up, fashioning a tube out of it. He will cut the gortex to the size he believes will best suit your heart, and then sew the gortex conduit into place on your heart." Dr. Stone explained this very slowly and drew out pictures as he spoke, making sure all of us understood what was going to happen.

A few weeks later my parents and I made the familiar trip down to Minneapolis Children's Hospital for another open heart surgery. We arrived just before 6:00 A.M. and walked into the lobby of the hospital. Once again I was amazed by the number of people waiting in the lobby of the hospital to see me before I went into surgery. The walls were lined with family members and friends, including dozens and dozens of high school students who woke up before 5:00 A.M. and arranged carpools in order to come to the hospital to be there for me. I was able to stop in the lobby and visit with everyone before I had to go back into the pre-op waiting area.

While I waited in my hospital bed for the surgery to begin, Dr. Stone came in to say hi to everyone and to go over the final plans of the surgery with us. Sensing that the time before surgery was running low, my brothers hugged me and began to cry. Tommy's 6'2" frame absolutely smothered me when he leaned over to hug me. His broad shoulders heaved up and down as he cried. I patted his back and tried to reassure him that everything was going to be all right. David was next in line, and once again was unable to say a single word through his tears. I rubbed his back and told him everything was going to work out just fine.

As my brothers stepped back, my parents came next to my bed to give me a hug. My dad squeezed my foot, and then leaned down and wrapped his arms around me. He whispered into my ear, "I love you, Bud. I love you." Then he stood back and rubbed my mom's back as she leaned over me. She was crying heavily and leaned in close to me. She grabbed me by the arm, looked me straight in the face, and said, "Nick, I didn't forget what you told me last time about not being worried about surgery, because it's just another day. But it's so hard not worry, I am just so scared. I wouldn't know what to do without you," she cried.

"It's okay," I said, trying to console her. "It's okay to be afraid, but understand I don't believe my life is in any greater risk today then I was in yesterday. God is in control of when we live and die. I will be here until I have done everything I have come to do. I just hope my work is a long way from being complete."

As my mom stood back up the nurse entered the room to bring me into surgery. I waved goodbye to everyone, told them I was going to go take a nap, and that I would see them in a little bit. I fell asleep staring at the ceiling tiles rushing past as I was being wheeled into the operating room.

As I began to come to after the surgery, both Tommy and David were at my bedside. Soon my parents and my grandma were in my room. My eyes wandered and jumped around the room as I struggled to focus on any single object.

"Nick, Honey, everything is okay. The surgery is done, and you did so good. Everyone is so proud of you." I heard my mom's voice, but I was unable to focus on her face.

"Bud, everything went well. We are all here with you now. Everything went great. Dr. Nicoloff said he was able to put the gortex piece in without any problems," my dad said while he was rubbing my arm.

I drifted in and out of consciousness as the anesthesia wore down. My eyes snapped wide open as people began to talk, but then squinted close as I drifted back to sleep.

"Nick, we will stay right here, Honey, just close your eyes and try to sleep a little more. Don't try and fight the anesthesia, just relax and sleep a while longer," my mom whispered to me.

As I became more aware of my surroundings, and more awake, the anesthesiologist came into my room. He talked with my nurse for a while in the corner of my room, and then walked alongside my bed.

"Nick, how are you feeling?" he asked. "I am going to remove the breathing tube from your throat. It looks like you are breathing pretty much on your own now, and having that tube out will really make you feel better."

As he spoke, he put on a pair of rubber gloves and began removing the tape around my mouth that was holding the tube in place.

"Okay, Nick, when I tell you to, I want you to take in a deep breath and hold it. When I remove the tube I want you to try to push all of the air out of your lungs. Do you understand?" he asked.

I nodded my head as I extended my hand to my mom who was sitting next to my bed. He began giving instructions to my nurse, and then he unhooked the tubing from the respirator connected to the tube in my throat. "Nick, go ahead and take in that deep breath, and one, two, three, breathe all the way out," he ordered.

I followed his directions closely, and coughed hard as I felt the end of the tube rise up my trachea and past the back of my throat, triggering my gag reflex.

"Good job. See, that wasn't so bad, and now your throat will feel much better," he said as I continued coughing and gagging.

Within a few hours of having the breathing tube removed I was sitting at a slight incline in bed, drinking little sips of apple juice, and visiting with my family. Within a few days I was transferred out of the Intensive Care Unit. A few days later I was discharged from Children's hospital, less then one week after my surgery.

After I was released from the hospital I continued my recovery at home. My teachers from the high school came to my home and visited with me. All of them were extremely helpful keeping me caught up with my coursework. Even though I missed over a month and a half of my junior year in high school, I was able to complete all of my assignments.

Once I started back at school it took a few weeks to get back in the swing of things. Soon, however, my energy level had returned to normal and I was able to resume my hectic high school routine. That spring, as juniors began deciding on their class schedules for their final year in high school, I decided to run for senior class president. I had always enjoyed being involved in extra-curricular activities throughout junior high and high school. The more I visited with other students in my class, the more I wanted to become president. The campaign stretched out for several weeks, and concluded with me being elected senior class president.

The last big event of the year was our Junior Prom. A large group of my friends all went to the dinner and dance together, and we had a fabulous time. I felt fantastic all night long and spent almost the entire evening on the dance floor. We all danced and partied, and just really had a lot of fun. After the dance we went to an after prom party where we ate even more food, visited, and watched movies until breakfast time.

It was no surprise how tired I was following that evening. Soon after prom I got run down with a cold, and didn't feel well. This continued a few weeks as the school year came to an end.

A week after school was out for the summer my mom came into my bedroom early in the morning to wake me up. She walked into my room, turned on my lights, and began telling me I needed to wake up.

"Nick! Nick, come on, get up! Tommy just called. He and Karla are on their way to the hospital. Karla is in labor; we need to get going, Nick." Her voiced seemed really loud as I tried to focus on what she was saying.

"Okay...okay," I mumbled as I climbed out of bed and headed towards the bathroom.

"Hurry up and hop in the shower! Tommy would be so disappointed if you missed his girl being born, especially since you missed the birth of his first daughter," my mom said.

I started the shower and went to the bathroom, still trying to clear my head and fully wake up. I climbed into the shower and quickly washed my hair and cleaned up. In the shower I felt so tired it seemed like everything I did was in slow motion. When I finished showering I dried off as quickly as I could and threw on some clean clothes. I quickly brushed my teeth, combed my hair, and shaved. As I finished up in the bathroom I fought the unbelievably strong urge to climb back in bed and go to sleep.

As I walked upstairs my mom was waiting in the entry ready to leave. I walked passed her, through the kitchen into the living room, and sat down on the couch. My dad walked into the living room from their bedroom and began speaking to me.

"Good morning, sleepy head," he said with a quirky smile. "What are your plans for tonight? Are you getting together with the guys?"

I turned my head to the left as he began to speak. I stared intently at him, watching his mouth move and hearing noise coming from him. However, no matter how hard I tried to focus, I couldn't understand any of the words he was saying. I was so confused. My dad was speaking, but it didn't even sound like English. I tried to listen harder, but still nothing he was saying made any sense to me at all.

My dad glanced down at me and noticed me silently staring at him. He walked closer to the couch, and repeated himself. "Nick, what are your plans for this evening? Are you hanging out with the guys?"

Still unable to understand any of the sounds coming from his mouth, I asked him to repeat what he said. When I tried to open my mouth to speak my tongue wouldn't cooperate with me. "Wha...Whaaaa...Whaa..." emanated from my mouth.

My mom was now standing behind my dad in the living room. I could see her face tense up, and a look of worry consumed her. My dad walked closer to me, still speaking. Although I could not understand what he was saying, I knew he was upset. He put his hands on my shoulder and under my elbow and began picking me up. "Come on, Bud, stand up," he said, in denial of what was going on.

As he pulled me up, the entire weight of my body fell forward because I was unable to support any weight on my own. I fell between the coffee table and the couch onto the floor, and rolled onto my back. I stared up at the ceiling as my dad quickly knelt beside me. He was shouting to my mother, and trying to talk to me. He put his hand in each of my hands, and motioned for me to squeeze his hands. I acknowledged what he wanted me to do, and I squeezed my hands into fists.

I watched the expression on his face drop, and he motioned to me over and over again to squeeze with my right hand. I tilted my head slightly down, and watched my left hand squeeze around my dad's fingers. Then I turned my head slightly, squeezed with my right hand, and watched as nothing happened.

My dad shifted down my body to my legs, and pressed his hands against my feet. He motioned for me to push with my legs. Again I watched my left foot move and press down against his hand. Then I looked at my right foot, and noticed it had remained in the same spot, completely motionless. My heart sunk, and tears began to roll down my cheeks. I realized that I had a stroke, and the entire right side of my body was paralyzed.

Within minutes the paramedics had arrived and began going over the same assessments my dad had done earlier. I couldn't tell them I had already tried to move my right arm and leg. I wept as they asked me to squeeze with my right hand,

and nothing happened. I began to panic when they asked me to press down with my right foot, and it still wouldn't move.

I looked up and saw my mom with a look of despair as the paramedics shifted me onto a backboard and lifted me onto the gurney. As the paramedics carried me out of the house my dad put his arm around my mom, and they walked out to the ambulance with the paramedics.

As I lay in the back of the ambulance staring at the ceiling, I could hear the paramedics talking. I grew more and more upset listening to them talk, not being able to understand what they were saying. Soon I could feel the ambulance accelerate, and I heard the siren blaring as the ambulance rocketed down the highway. During the trip in the ambulance I stared down at my right hand and right foot, trying to make them move. I couldn't believe that I was still unable to move or feel the right side of my body.

I stopped trying to move my arm and leg, and just closed my eyes and cried. I was absolutely devastated that I was paralyzed. I quickly became very angry that this had happened. I was so mad that after everything I had been through, now I was going to be trapped in a paralyzed body, unable to communicate with anyone. I thought to myself, Seven open heart surgeries, two years waiting for a heart transplant, and now, after making it through all that, I won't even be able to wipe my own ass.

Dr. Stone was waiting for the ambulance in the emergency room at Minneapolis Children's Hospital. When the paramedics wheeled me into a room in the ER I saw Dr. Stone's face drop. While the nurses began to get me settled in the ER, I began to recover some of my senses. Slowly I was beginning to understand more and more of what people around me were saying. Soon after I arrived, my speech began to return, although it was obviously slurred. A few minutes later my parents arrived, and began talking to Dr. Stone and the neurologist.

"Nick, we just talked to the doctors," my mom said in a voice that was obviously designed to be comforting. "They are going to run some tests, but they think they may be able to fix any damage done by this. They are hoping this is all just temporary, and that after a while everything will be okay."

"Bud," my dad began, "no matter what happens, we are going to make it through this. We have all been through too much to let this screw anything up. No matter what happens, everything will be all right. We will figure this out. We have to make it through this. We will make it through this," he repeated.

After the neurologist spoke with the emergency room nurse I was quickly taken to radiology for a CT scan. The results of the scan showed that I had indeed suffered a minor trans-ischemic attack, or a mild stroke. The small clot had lodged in a blood vessel in my brain for a few moments and then kept traveling. The neurologist immediately ordered the nurses to administer a new drug that was designed to breakup blood clots causing strokes. Several hours after this medication was given to me, improvement was rapid and dramatic. Steadily the movement in the right side of my body continued to improve, and my speech began to clear up.

Later that afternoon my dad and I were sitting in my hospital room watching television, trying to forget about the day. My mom walked into the room and shook her head. "Well, that's two nieces you've missed being born because you were in the hospital. I just can't believe something happened like this so unexpectedly. I guess maybe we have to tell your brother not to have anymore kids," she joked.

Although my recovery from the stroke was very quick, the doctors still didn't know why I had the stroke. Dr. Stone ran several tests throughout the rest of the summer, trying to determine how and where the blood clot could have formed in my body. Blood pooling and potentially clotting in my legs was quickly ruled out as a source of the stroke. Several tests and a scan of my lungs ruled out additional clots in my lungs.

Finally, in late summer, an angiogram revealed what Dr. Stone had been dreading all along. Blood was leaking in between the gortex conduit on the right side of my heart and the left atrium. The mixing of the blood explained all of my symptoms of fatigue before the stroke, and probably played a role in the formation of the blood clot. By studying the X-ray films of the radioactive dye migrating through my heart, Dr. Stone was able to determine that a stitch holding the gortex conduit to the heart muscle had come loose. This opening allowed a small amount of blood to move back and forth between the two sides of the heart. This news devastated my parents and me, because we all knew this meant yet another open heart surgery.

A New Stroke
Of Fortune

A few months after my stroke, as summer was beginning to come to an end, I met someone who would change my life forever. During the month of August the Elk River High School student council met to organize the homecoming celebration that occurs just a few weeks into school. At that meeting I met Julie Pearson-Roden. Julie was an incoming sophomore student council representative. During that daylong meeting I was able to visit with Julie and get to know her.

At the end of the day, I looked for Julie, hoping to visit more. I could not find her anywhere. She had left and all I could think about as I left the high school was talking to her again. When I got home I looked in the phone book for her number. I never imagined how hard it could be to find someone with a hyphenated name! After talking to an uncle of hers, I finally had her number. Only, our first phone conversation did not go as easily as I had planned.

Ring…ring…ring. I waited patiently for her to answer.

"Hello?" Julie answered.

"Hi Julie, this is Nick Zerwas. We met at the student council meeting today…you probably are sur—"

"Hello? Hello? Is anyone there? I'm sorry, but I can't hear you, you'll have to call back!" Julie explained regretfully.

What? I wondered, was this a joke? My voice may be soft, but I have never had anyone actually hang up on me because they could not hear me. I called back and again was hung up on, and on the third call, I made more progress.

"Hi, Nick. I am really sorry, I can hardly hear you...the phone is acting up and all I hear is a buzzing noise," Julie said, embarrassed.

"Oh. Well I was wondering if maybe you wanted to do something tonight. I was going to be with my friends, but apparently their plans were for a couples night, so I thought maybe we could go to a movie or something."

"Okay, come on over," she said, and proceeded to give me directions to her house.

During the last few weeks of summer vacation Julie and I became inseparable. Julie already knew about my heart problem, but she never seemed to dwell on it. She was always so happy and positive; I just felt better when I was around her.

My senior year at Elk River High School began just a few days after I learned that I would need to have another surgery. The first few months of the school year passed very quickly as my parents and I worked with Dr. Stone and Dr. Nicoloff to schedule the surgery. Dr. Nicoloff studied fancy systems of using a prefabricated patch that would expand on both sides of the hole in my heart and eventually be grown over by tissue. However, he determined the unique physiology of my heart would complicate the procedure too much. He decided the only way to repair the gortex was to open my chest once again, and re-stitch the tiny hole closed.

After I found out about the impending surgery, I put off telling Julie for several weeks. However, it didn't take her long to realize something was wrong and that I was acting differently. After another appointment with Dr. Stone, I went back up to the high school to catch Julie before she went to soccer practice.

I got there just as she was heading down to the locker room and asked her to sit at one of the lunch tables. I felt nervous, like the times I had told my parents I knew something was wrong. I didn't want to scare Julie away, make her worry, or change anything between us. Everything had been going so well, and I was scared to lose her. I knew that she was different, though, and somehow knew that she would understand. I explained to her that at my appointment, surgery was scheduled to repair the mixing blood in my heart. She asked questions about how serious it was, and how I felt, but she never got upset. She was concerned and compassionate, and made me feel supported. I told her not to worry and that we would talk more later, knowing that she had to get to practice. She teased me for telling her when she didn't have time to talk, to avoid those "mushy" feelings, and left, after a long hug and words of encouragement.

A few weeks later, one of Julie's friends, Adria Bykowski, had a group of us over for her birthday party. Knowing that my surgery was just a few weeks away, Julie and I made the most of the night by talking with everyone and playing games. After the party, I drove Julie home, and we sat in her driveway and talked.

"Nick, are you worried about your surgery? You keep saying you aren't, but how can you not be?" Julie questioned delicately.

"No I'm not worried...besides, what good would that do?" I chuckled, but then noticed her sad expression.

"Nick, it is okay to worry, anyone would before a surgery like this. If we want to stay together, we have to be honest with each other. You hiding your emotions only hurts me, and stops us from helping each other through this. This is hard, but we can't do it like this."

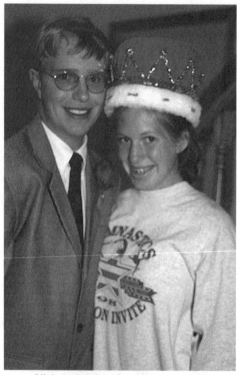

Nick and Julie after Homecoming
Nick's senior year

"I know. I'm sorry. It's just that I am not used to having someone that is not scared by this and I don't want to see you sad because of me," I tried to explain. "I mean, my whole life I have dealt with things as they came and accepted them, with my family always beside me, but I have never had anyone I felt this way about involved."

"I know, but now you do. So let's be together and start talking. I won't be sad as long as you are honest with me. I know you have been through a lot, but I am here with you and your family now, so let's all stick together," Julie concluded.

"I know, I know," I whispered back to her.

The surgery was scheduled for Thanksgiving break, in order to allow me to miss the least amount of class as possible. That morning when we arrived at Minneapolis Children's Hospital, I was greeted by a familiar and comforting scene. The entire lobby of the hospital was filled with my family members, friends, and loved ones. Again, entire carloads of students made the trip down to Minneapolis at 5:00 A.M. I was able to greet everyone who had come to wish me well and support my family. There was a new addition to this pre-surgery routine, and that was my girlfriend of several months, Julie. Julie, along with my family, was at my side before surgery.

In the moments before I was taken into surgery, my family went through our usual routine of hugs, tears, and words of encouragement. After I said my good-byes to my brothers and parents, I hugged Julie closely and told her I would see her in a little while.

Several weeks later I had returned to school, and my focus quickly shifted away from recovering from surgery and on to preparing for graduation. My parents and I had thought of that day often, but on many occasions never believed we would ever make it to that point. As the time drew nearer I grew more appreciative of the realization that I was actually going to graduate from high school. I had made it through eight open heart surgeries, I had waited for a heart transplant in the hospital for nearly six months, I had recovered from a stroke that had initially left me unable to move or speak the year before. Now, finally, the time had arrived.

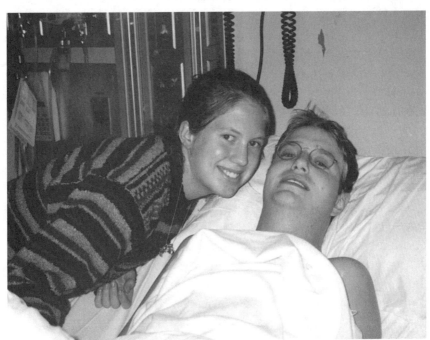

Nick and Julie after Nick's senior year surgery (winter 1998)

"Okay, it's done. I hope everyone likes it," I said cheerfully.

"Oh, Nick, it's awesome. People are going to love it," my dad said, beaming.

"I can't believe it was right in front of me everyday. I must have read that a thousand times, but now I truly appreciate what it means," I told my parents. I gave them both a big hug, and thanked them for all their help.

That morning my mom ironed my black graduation gown, while I fiddled with my graduation cap in the mirror. "Mom, are you sure this thing is on right? I look kinda goofy," I joked.

"Nick, it looks perfect. You look great," she said with a smile.

After my gown was pressed and on, and I had rearranged my cap a hundred more times, we all went outside to take photos. Julie and I took a few photos before she had to go to the high school to warm-up with the band. Everyone took turns posing next to me, and then my brothers picked me up and held me up high for one final photo. When we arrived at the school my parents dropped me off so I could go around to the other side of the gymnasium and get into line with my friends. Since I was the senior class president, I was given a reserved spot at the beginning of the line. This meant I was going to lead the class into the gym and be the first student to receive a diploma.

As the band began playing the graduation march, I was given the signal by Mr. Voight, the principal, to begin walking. We wound around the corner and into the packed room. I looked up and smiled as I walked down the center of the aisle. I spotted my family sitting in the first row along the bleachers next to the stage, and Julie over in the band. As I sat down my knees shook a little bit as I glanced at the speech I was about to read.

A few minutes later Mr. Voight introduced me to the audience, and I climbed the stairs onto the stage. I shook his hand, and took my place behind the podium. I glanced around the gym packed with people, and glanced down to my parents and smiled. I leaned forward so my voice could be heard throughout the room, and I began.

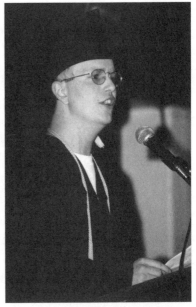

Nick giving graduation speech

Good evening, everyone, and thank you all for coming tonight to honor and celebrate the graduation of the class of 1999.

To the class of 1999, I would like you to remember that, yesterday is history, tomorrow is a mystery, and today is a gift…that's why it is called the present.

That saying has been on my refrigerator door at home for a very long time. I have read it many times and thought about it an awful lot.

Yesterday is history. What we have done in the past, good or bad, is now behind us. So, do not dwell on your past mistakes or gloat too long on your victories, because yesterday is history.

Tomorrow is a mystery. What will tomorrow bring? Good news or bad, sickness or good health? Don't waste a day of living worrying about what tomorrow will bring—tomorrow is a mystery.

The gift we have is today, the present. Each day we wake up is a gift, something never to be wasted.

The class of 1999 can change the world. We can change the world by never wasting the gift of each day we are given.

If we use everyday to the best of our ability we will change the world. "How?" you ask. Very simply, in small ways, like smiling at a handicapped person instead of turning your face away.

By visiting your elderly neighbor, or helping someone who is ill. Each and every day we can make the world a nicer place by doing something as simple as smiling.

If everyone of us did just one act of kindness each and every day, think of the difference we could make.

Not all of us are going to end up being rocket scientists or curing cancer, but that doesn't mean each one of us can't make a difference in the world.

Let us, the class of 1999, make a pledge to change the world one day at a time by using our hearts. By doing our best with each day, each GIFT that is given to us, by never wasting a day worrying about yesterday or tomorrow, by living and doing our best in the present. We will always have the hope of a brighter, happier tomorrow.

On behalf of the class of 1999, I would like to thank all of our parents, brothers, sisters, grandparents, godparents, aunts, uncles, and friends. You are all our community of love and support. We thank you all for helping us during our school years. You have helped us make it to this day of graduation.

A special thank you to all of our teachers, principals, and school staff from kindergarten, through this year. Your support, understanding, kindness, and most of all, your patience with us, is very much appreciated.

Graduates, let's give our families, friends, and school staff a heartfelt round of applause.

To all our classmates and loved ones who have passed away, including my grandfathers and my little buddy Blake, we know you are smiling down on us tonight. We are graduating for you, and we miss you.

Now, would everyone please stand up. Would just the class of 1999 please be seated. Now, please let the record reflect that the 1999 graduating class of Elk River High School received a well-deserved standing ovation.

Epilogue

I had a great summer after high school, filled with graduation parties and best friends saying their good-byes as they prepared to go their separate ways.

I chose to attend Hamline University because it was a small, beautiful campus where I could handle the walking distances between classes and get a great education. Hamline, located in St. Paul, Minnesota, was close enough to home, and of course, to Julie, my high school sweetheart, who still had two years of high school left.

My parents helped me move into my dorm room in late August with pride and fear. It was an emotional day for the entire Zerwas family, and another milestone in my life that had seemed hard to dream about for the first eighteen years of my life.

I was able to make many new friends quickly and enjoyed my new life as a college student. In my second month of school, however, I started feeling tired and very fatigued. Once again I made the phone call with the same dreaded words…"Dr. Stone, I don't feel well."

After taking a few tests and wearing a 24-hour halter monitor to record my heart rate and rhythm, Dr. Stone called me. "It's not good," he said with a sigh; he was always open and honest and never kept us in suspense. After knowing him for eighteen years, I could read his voice and body language. My heart rate at night had dropped to only 16 beats per minute. I needed a pacemaker right away.

Dr. Nicoloff, my surgeon, was in China. We decided to wait for his return in five days, and I was immediately hospitalized for the wait.

Surgery was complicated because of my previous surgeries and a great deal of scar tissue. Most people get a pacemaker as a short stay surgery, leaving the hospital the same day. My surgery, however, involved spreading my ribs to get behind my lungs and heart so the leads of the pacemaker could be attached to the back of my heart. There were complications—a lung collapsed and there was fluid in my diaphragm—and recovery took months. Still, I didn't miss a single semester of college. My professors, who had only known me for three months prior to surgery, called constantly to check on me and help me with all of my classes. I was able to complete my first semester of classes at Hamline without having to drop a single credit.

The next three and a half years flew by smoothly. Julie graduated from high school—in the top twenty, no less, besting my own high school ranking. She chose to attend the College of Saint Catherine and majored in nursing.

After graduating from Hamline, I decided to work in the Anoka County Sheriff's crime lab, where I had interned during college. The sheriff's office employees welcomed and looked after me as part of their law enforcement family.

On December 15, 2003, my 23rd birthday, I asked Julie Pearson-Roden to be my wife. We started planning a June 25, 2005, wedding.

I continued work at the Sheriff's office and began graduate school in education at Hamline University while Julie finished her education at the College of St. Catherine's.

In December of 2004, six months before our wedding, I had a scheduled check up. Dr. Stone was now retired, but still very much a part of my life. Dr. Stone chose his colleague, Dr. Sutton, to be my new cardiologist. Dr. Sutton had been a partner in the clinic with Dr. Stone since I had been an infant.

Julie, along with both of our parents, joined me for a routine checkup at the clinic. Within minutes after testing began on my pacemaker, Julie went to the waiting room and waved for my folks to join us. My pacemaker was not functioning. The lead had fractured and my heart was not being paced.

My surgeon, Dr. Nicoloff, who was the only surgeon who had touched my heart, had passed away just a few years earlier. It was hard to imagine another surgeon working on my heart, but there was no other choice.

Amazingly, the surgery went very well, with no complications, and I was home in just three days. Julie graduated in the spring, and just six months after my last surgery we were married. My big brothers were the best men and Julie's sister was the matron of honor. All of our friends,

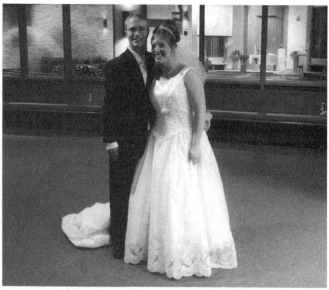

Nick and Julie, married June 25, 2005

family, and community supporters—including my mentor Dr. Frederic Stone, who read at the wedding ceremony—witnessed the moment in my life that no one ever dared to dream of. My high school sweetheart, Julie, and I were now Mr. and Mrs. Nicholas Howard Zerwas!

Everyone celebrated life, love, hope and faith. The prayers of my community supporters, family, wife, and myself, had been answered.

Order Form

Please copy this page, add the necessary information, and mail it with your check or money order, payable to Nick Zerwas to:

> Nick Zerwas
> 6956 139th Ave NW
> Ramsey MN 55303

ISBN: 1-930374-17-8
The Gift Of An Open Heart $18.00 each   Qty. _____

Total: _____

MN residents add 6.5% sales tax ($1.17/book) _____

Shipping: $2.00 first book, $1.00 each additional _____

Total enclosed: _____

Name: _____

Address: _____

City: _____ State: _____ Zip: _____

Phone: (__) _____ Email:_____

You can also order this book online at www.NickZerwas.com or from DeForest Press at www.DeForestPress.com. If you'd like to order by phone, call DeForest Press at 612-527-1623, or toll-free at 1-877-441-9733.